MEDICARE GOALZ 4 U

Your Guide to Enrolling in Medicare

TONI KING

Medicare Disclaimer:
This book/guide is not associated, endorsed, or authorized by the Social Security Administration, the Department of Health and Human Services or the Centers for Medicare & Medicaid Services. This book/guide contains basic information about Medicare, services related to Medicare and services for Medicare beneficiaries. If you would like more information about the Federal Government's Medicare program, please visit the office U.S. Government's site for Medicare beneficiaries located at www.medicare.gov.

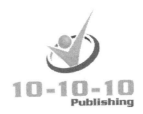

10-10-10
Publishing

Medicare Goalz 4 U – Your Guide to Enrolling in Medicare

www.tonisays.com

Copyright © 2019 Toni King

ISBN: 978-0-578-48453-2

Publisher
10-10-10 Publishing
Markham, ON
Canada

Printed in the United States and in Canada.

DEDICATION

I wish to dedicate this book to my weekly, nationwide Medicare column readers, whose various Medicare questions have helped to write this book, to help America understand how confusing enrolling in Medicare can be. The Toni Says® Medicare readers have made me realize that America is more confused about how to enroll in Medicare than Washington, D.C. is aware.

Most of all, I give thanks to God for placing the passion in my heart to help America understand what should be a simple governmental system, but only seems to be getting more complicated as more Americans are enrolling in Medicare.

TESTIMONIALS

1."I'd like to thank you for your incredible expertise..."

Dear Toni,

I'd like to thank you for your incredible expertise in helping me to understand the confusing world of Medicare. I have been following your articles in a local community newspaper for many years, so when it came time for me to sign up for Medicare, I knew just the right person to contact. You are awesome! Due to your thorough knowledge of Medicare, and with your guidance, I have a complete feeling of peace, knowing that I am enrolled in the appropriate Medicare Plans for me. Your passion and mission in helping others is a true gift to everyone you have helped over the years. God bless you!

Sally

2."...thank Toni for her dedication and for all the hard work..."

Hello *Toni Says*,

I just wanted to thank Toni for her dedication and for all the hard work that she does to help people like me sort through this Social Security and Medicare stuff. I am so thankful for everything that Toni does, and for all of you who help her do what is necessary to help us get through the paperwork. I just wanted to let Toni know that I have recently been diagnosed with a rare blood disorder, and I am currently taking a chemo pill for this disorder. I've had many doctor visits (I see 3 doctors), and many tests. Because of the help you gave me to choose the Medicare supplements, my doctors and meds have been very affordable. Even the chemo meds are under $30, and that is a 90-day supply! Things could have been so much worse. I thank God for His love and mercy, and His wisdom to send me to you. I can't thank you enough.

Please keep up the good work. There are so many people who need you, and you have been a wonderful blessing to so many!

Love,

Kary from Houston, TX

3."You have always been there for us, to guide us through the maze."

Hi Toni,

I know you're working on updating your website, but I wanted to share our testimonial of how much you have helped my wife and me with both Social Security and Medicare. Please feel free to post this in your "What People Are Saying….."

All that planning paid off when it finally came time for us to initially file for Social Security, and last year for Medicare. We soon found out that when it came to Medicare Medi-Gap insurance and prescription services, you always looked out for what was best for us.

But as with anything you do for the first time, there was a lot of worrying that we had overlooked a minor detail that would live with us for the rest of our retirement. We had watched our parents manage to barely get by with their

Social Security benefits, and struggle with the changes in medical care as they began their lives with Medicare.

But you have always been there for us, to guide us through the maze. I saw where someone recently said you're the Zen Master of Medicare, and you are. And even when we'd completed the forms correctly, and we just needed your assurance that we'd done it right, you were always there. Almost like the woobie blanket from Mr. Mom.

Thank you so much!

John S

4."I can assure you that without your knowledge and expertise, I would have been lost..."

Dear Toni:

I am writing this letter to thank you for all your help when I was searching for an insurance company to replace my old policy that had been dropped by my doctor's office.

In order to continue to use my doctor, I had no choice but to find another insurance company that my doctor would accept.

I can assure you that without your knowledge and expertise, I would have been lost in finding an insurance company that had the benefits that I needed. Again, I want to thank you for your advice and guidance, and to let you know how pleased I am with my new insurance company.

Very truly yours,

Loy M

CONTENTS

FOREWORD

The U.S. is reaching a crossroads, as the biggest generation, a.k.a. the Baby Boomers, are reaching the age of 65. This generation is aging and that means the Medicare enrollment numbers are going to swell over the next decade. For those who are getting ready to 65, *Medicare Goalz 4 U – The Guide to Enrolling in Medicare* is a must!

Toni King has decades of experience working as a Medicare enrollment consultant, helping people to navigate this complicated government program. For those in the U.S., enrolling in Medicare is a reality for a majority of Americans once they turn 65. However, there is also plenty of confusing information out there, being spread by well-meaning friends, family, and co-workers that can end up costing you thousands of dollars.

Part of the message of *Medicare Goalz 4 U – The Guide to Enrolling in Medicare* is to help you understand when you need to enroll in Medicare and dispel some of that erroneous information along the way. You will learn about the initial enrollment period at your 65th birthday, if you qualify to delay your Medicare benefits without any penalties, and the potential impact of a late enrollment in Medicare.

As part of this guide, Toni also provides Goalz 4 U at the end of each chapter, summarizing key points and giving you a checklist to help throughout your enrollment process. Do not go off the information you received from co-workers or family members. Get this guide and give yourself the information you need to successfully navigate enrolling in Medicare!

Raymond Aaron
New York Bestselling Author

Introduction

Medicare brings to mind the golden years when you and your sweetheart are retired, and now life is supposed to be peachy-keen and wonderful. Your health is taken care of, and there is nothing to worry about. Wrong!!

I am Toni King, and my goal is to help those new to the Medicare system understand the process, starting from enrollment. I want to put you back in control of your Medicare health care. Most of all, it will help YOUR Social Security and retirement check—what you worked so hard for! How did I get involved in Medicare and helping others? It all started one Saturday morning in January 2008. I was working with Mr. Davis, assisting him in straightening out a problem he had encountered, which was caused by a misguided Social Security employee that nearly kept him from receiving his Medicare Part B.

After I saw how confused he was with the Medicare system, I decided that I needed to write a simple guide to help the average person understand how to enroll in the maze of Medicare. That guide became my book, *The Medicare Survival Guide Advanced*, available at www.tonisays.com. I will reference that guide throughout this book, as it contains the additional information you need to make smart coverage choices once you enroll in Medicare.

Every day, I work with those on Medicare, who think that Social Security and Medicare will take care of them. Seniors are dog paddling to keep their noses above water and stay afloat, trying to pay their medical and prescription drug bills, not to mention the lights, water, phone, and so much more. The bills are not going down but are headed straight up! If you are not on top of your enrollment, it can mean having to stretch your dollars even further.

I am passionate about helping our aging population access the benefits that they have paid for throughout their working life. Plus, America's Medicare population is set to increase as 10,000 Baby Boomers a day turn 65! Perhaps you are not one of those Baby Boomers, but you have a parent who is set to turn 65, or is older. Regardless of your situation, all of us are going to be impacted by Medicare enrollment at some point.

Medicare is available to all Americans once they reach 65. However, enrolling can feel like working through an Escape Room. After all, you don't know what you don't know, but those things can end up coming back to bite you regarding your Medicare enrollment.

The information contained in this book is critical to making sure that you are addressing all aspects of enrolling in Medicare. I call them Goalz 4 U, and each *goalz* is critical to taking the right steps throughout the process.

By using this enrollment guide as you begin this journey, you can avoid those mistakes that can end up costing you financially, at a time when you need medical insurance or prescription drug coverage to assist you in paying for expenses related to addressing chronic medical conditions or major life-threatening emergencies. That is not the time to find out that you are responsible for a larger financial piece of the pie, or worse, to find out that you are not covered at all!

The fact is that Medicare can be confusing, particularly the enrollment process. I have been working in this industry for decades. Time and again, I meet individuals who did not follow through on delaying their Medicare Parts A, B, or D properly, only to find themselves struggling to deal with requirements for Medicare that can negatively impact your monthly Medicare premiums with Medicare Parts B and/or D penalties, putting you at financial risk, particularly if you are retired and on a fixed income.

It can be easy to get confused when enrolling in Medicare at 65 or after 65, for a variety of reasons such as:

Are you turning 65 and receiving your Social Security check? Different ways to enroll.

Are you turning 65, receiving your Social Security check, and enrolled in your spouse's (who is working full-time) company group health benefits? Different ways to enroll.

Are you turning 65, not receiving your Social Security check, and not working full-time with company benefits? Different ways to enroll.

Are you turning 65, not receiving your Social Security check, working full-time with no company benefits, and maybe have an individual plan or VA benefits? Different ways to enroll.

Are you past 65, retiring from your current employment, and never enrolled in Medicare Parts A and/or B? Different ways to enroll.

There are so many myths and half-truths out there that I could write a whole book just on those alone. One of the biggest mistakes that people make is taking information from a family member, a friend, or even a doctor or HR employee, and believing it is accurate. As you can tell, there is a lot of information out there, but very little of it is on point. I want you to be aware of the myths and misinformation, so you can make smart choices and avoid the confusing traps.

This process is more complicated than many individuals realize. It is not always automatic, and even though you have paid into the system for years, there is no guarantee that you will get the coverage that fits your needs if you make a mistake during the enrollment process. In fact, you could end up sabotaging yourself.

Another point to keep in mind is that no matter what anyone tells you, including the individuals at the Social Security office, verbal information means nothing. You need hard copies of everything that you do with Social Security, which is where you will enroll for Medicare. I encourage everyone that I work with to make sure that you have copies of all paperwork, and that you put a copy in a backup location, along with all the other critical documents you need to keep safe, such as your Social Security card or other key pieces of identification.

Part of my job as a Medicare consultant and advocate is to work with you throughout the enrollment process, providing you the guidance necessary to make sure that you are not shooting your future self in the foot. That being said, I can't be everywhere. This book is meant to specifically address the potential traps involved in the process of enrollment. Once you enroll, then there are other choices to make regarding the various parts of Medicare. However, if you don't enroll properly, then it can impact what type of options you have, and the financial implications from those options.

Throughout the rest of the chapters of this book, I am going to focus on helping you to understand what Medicare is, and what its basic options are. After giving you a rundown of Medicare, I want to focus in on enrollment periods. This part is critical, because individuals often misunderstand how this period works, thus leaving them in a precarious position. Finally, I am going to focus in on different scenarios, and give you the information you need to successfully handle your Medicare enrollment, regardless of your situation.

At the end of each chapter, I am also going to include Goalz 4 U, which will give you a quick guide of critical points to remember from each chapter. There are also going to be references to various forms, and I have included pictures of what the forms look like, in Chapter 9, so you know exactly what you need to have. As always, you can contact me for consultations, and address your questions, at my website, www.tonisays.com, or by email, at info@tonisays.com.

By the end of this book, I want you to understand when you need to enroll, where you are going to enroll, why you need to enroll, and how to enroll. I want to give you the tools necessary to successfully answer all these questions, regardless of your personal situation.

Let's get started!

GOALZ 1
Understanding Medicare ABC&D

Medicare is a government-controlled insurance program that every American can qualify for, thus giving them medical care coverage when turning 65, during retirement, or if they are unable to work before 65 due to a disability. In a world where medical costs continue to rise, and for retirees, their income often does not, Medicare provides a safety net to help them address their various medical issues. We all deal with them as we age, and some of those chronic conditions and the medications used to treat them can have a huge financial impact.

However, Medicare is not just one insurance plan that covers everything. It is divided into parts, often known as Medicare Part A, Part B, Part C, and Part D. Each of these parts cover a specific aspect of your medical care. When you are choosing various aspects of Medicare Part A, Part B, Part C, and Part D, it is important to understand what is covered and what is not. Tailoring your Medicare choices can be done based on who you have as doctors, what your health conditions are, what types of medications you take, and what they cost.

There is a lot to consider as you begin the enrollment process. So, let's find out exactly what is covered when you are enrolled in Medicare, and what requires you to pay premiums. I want to start with Part A and what it covers.

What is Part A? (Hospital Insurance)

Medicare Part A is the in-hospital part of Original Medicare. Most people do not have to pay for Medicare Part A. You or your spouse must have worked at least 10 years (*40 quarters*), paying into the social security system, to receive Medicare Part A premium-free.

Toni Says®: *Usually, Medicare Part A begins the first day of the month you turn 65 and are enrolled in Medicare, or the 25th month if you are under 65 and receiving Social Security benefits. For those not receiving Social Security benefits and "is still working" with company benefits prior to turning 65, you must go online to* **www.ssa.gov/ benefits/medicare,** *3 months prior to turning 65, and enroll in Medicare to be sure your Medicare begins the month you turn 65. This is Very Important!!* ****Those still working with an HSA may consider not enrolling in Medicare due to the fact that even if you are enrolled in Medicare Part A, you can no long fund your HSA**** More on what Medicare Part A covers, in the Medicare Survival Guide® Advanced edition, which is available at www.tonisays.com.

Still, you may have questions regarding what Medicare Part A covers. After all, despite what its name implies, there is more covered than just in-patient hospital stays. For instance, if you have a surgery, a skilled nursing stay, or need blood, that is covered under Medicare Part A. Your chronic condition might require home health care or hospice. If that is the case, then it will be covered under Medicare Part A.

Depending on your health needs, there are other areas that Medicare Part A covers, as you can see below:

What does Part A Pay for?

- Blood
- Home Health Care
- Hospice Care

- In-patient Hospital Stay
- Skilled Nursing Facility

What is <u>MEDICARE PART B</u>? (Medical Insurance)

Medicare Part B pays for medically necessary services, such as doctors' services, office visits, doctor performing surgery, outpatient hospital care, and home health care that Medicare Part A does not cover. It also helps pay for some preventive services *("some" but not all preventive services)*. Clearly, this part is key to covering your regular health care, be it physicals or maintenance for chronic conditions. I have included more on what Medicare Part B covers, in the Medicare Survival Guide® Advanced edition, which is available by going to www.tonisays.com.

Now, it is important to recognize that while you might not have premiums for Medicare Part A, you are going to have a premium deducted for Medicare Part B. This premium can be deducted from your social security check, but if you are not collecting your social security, you will have to pay a monthly premium, as you pay for health insurance now.

I also want to be clear that your premium is not frozen at one price. In fact, it is going to change from year to year. Therefore, you need to be prepared for premium adjustments. Now, you might be deciding to NOT TAKE Medicare Part B, for a variety of reasons. For instance, you might think that the premium is out of the reach of your budget, or you might be thinking, "I don't get sick." These are not reasons to avoid enrolling in Medicare Part B.

There are no exceptions to the enrolling process for Medicare Part B, so make sure when you are ready to get on Medicare that you enroll and take Medicare Part B. This is especially important if you are not working full-time, with an employer's group benefits, or if you are not covered by a working spouse. Even if you are covered by these alternatives, it is important to follow the documentation process to avoid being hit with a penalty when you take Medicare down the road.

The Medicare Part B penalty is a 10% penalty per 12-month period that you could have had Medicare Part B but chose not to enroll or take it. This penalty is not limited to a specific timeframe but must be paid in addition to your monthly premium for the rest of your life. You can see how quickly this could get very expensive. After one year, the penalty is 10%, but after 3 years, it is up to 30%, and so on. Therefore, it is key that you document your reasons for delaying Medicare Part B, doing so according to the regulations of Social Security.

Toni Says: Usually, Medicare Part B begins the first day of the month you turn 65 and are enrolled in Medicare, or the 25th month if you are under 65 and receiving Social Security benefits. For those not receiving Social Security benefits prior to turning 65, you must go to Social Security 3 months prior to turning 65, and enroll in Medicare, or go online at **www.ssa.gov/benefits/ medicare** to be sure your Medicare Part B begins the month you turn 65. This is Very Important!!

There is a variety of expenses covered under Medicare Part B. It includes the doctors or surgeons that you may have to use as part of a hospital visit, or during your regular medical care. Here are a few of the other things covered under Medicare Part B.

What does Part B pay for?

- <u>Medical and Other Services</u> (Example: outpatient surgery, surgeon, doctor visits, anesthesiologist, pathologists, second surgical opinion, etc.).

- <u>Clinical Laboratory Services</u>

- <u>Home Health Care</u>

- <u>Durable Medical Equipment and Other Services</u>

- <u>Blood</u>

*Note – One more important thing for you to remember is that doctors or suppliers must agree to accept Medicare Assignment. This assignment means that the patient will not be required to pay any expense in excess of Medicare's approved charge. For many patients, this can be a cost savings in terms of what you must pay out of pocket.

Now, at the same time, there may also be specific costs that you will have to cover under Medicare Part B. It is important to check with your medical facility or doctor to determine what will be covered and what is going to be your financial responsibility.

Then there are Medicare Advantage Plans to help pick up the out-of-pocket costs that Medicare Part A and B have. (Medicare Advantage and Medicare Supplement plans are not the same.)

<u>MEDICARE PART C</u> (Medicare Advantage Plan)

Medicare Part C is another way to get your Medicare benefits and have what Original/Traditional Medicare does not pay for, paid by the Medicare

Advantage Plan. There can be co-pays to pay, but Medicare Part C can help with your out-of-pocket expenses. Private insurance companies, approved by Medicare, manage Medicare Part C. These Medicare Advantage plans must cover medically necessary services, but can charge different co-payments, co-insurance, or deductibles for these services.

There are a variety of Medicare Advantage Plans available, and each of them has different pros and cons, depending on your medical needs. It is important to recognize that you need to review each of these plans to determine the one that will fit your needs. What is included in a Medicare Advantage Plan?

First, a Medicare Advantage Plan or Part C is a health plan option (HMO, PPO, PFFS, MSA & SNP), which is operated by a private insurance company. To access this coverage, you need to present your Medicare Advantage Insurance Card, not your Medicare card.

It is also important to note that an Advantage Plan is not the same as a Medicare Supplement Plan. They cover different aspects of care at different rates, and this could impact your out-of-pocket costs. Also keep in mind the following:

- A MAPD plan provides your Medicare Part A *(hospital insurance)* and Medicare Part B *(medical insurance)* medically necessary services that Original/Traditional Medicare Plan provides.

- MAPD plans charge copayments, coinsurance, and deductibles for all services.

- MAPD Plans offer extra benefits that Original Medicare does not offer, such as vision, hearing, dental, diet, and exercise programs.

- Most Medicare Advantage Plans have a network of providers.

Reader Alert: CHECK WITH YOUR HOSPITAL AND DOCTOR BEFORE YOU ATTEMPT TO ENROLL IN A PART C MEDICARE ADVANTAGE PLAN. FIND OUT IF THEY ACCEPT THE PLAN YOU ARE CHOOSING!

Finally, there is the Part D of Medicare, which addresses another area where your costs can be impacted.

MEDICARE PART D (Medicare Prescription Drug Plan)

Medicare Part D helps cover prescription drugs and can be especially important if you are dealing with chronic conditions that require multiple prescriptions to address your symptoms. This coverage helps to lower your prescription drug costs. You are only required to have Medicare Part A to be eligible for a Medicare Prescription Drug Plan.

Most people enroll in both Medicare Part A and Part B when they become eligible for Medicare, but some will wait until later to get Medicare Part D. There are many reasons for delaying Medicare Part D, such as having group benefits, still working, having VA benefits, and more. Medicare does not force you to enroll in a Medicare Prescription Drug Plan. However, if you fail to enroll when you are first eligible, you will face a penalty of 1% per month that you wait to enroll.

You can only change your Medicare Advantage or Medicare Part D plan during Medicare Open/Annual Enrollment from October 15th to December 7th every year, which Medicare calls the Annual Enrollment Period (aka Open Enrollment). This enrollment period allows you to make changes to the plan you might have previously chosen, as well as enroll if you had previously delayed enrolling in Medicare Part D. Let's say you wait 3 years or 36 months to enroll in a Medicare Prescription Drug Plan. You will pay a **PENALTY** of 36 months x 1% = 36% more for as long as you are on Medicare. Don't wait!

Here is what you need to know about Medicare Part D Plans. First, there are two ways to enroll, such as a stand-alone with original Medicare and a Medicare Supplement, or with original Medicare only. You can also enroll in a Medicare Part D along with your Medicare Advantage Plan, known as a MAPD.

Drug Tiers include:

- Tier 1 – Preferred Generic
- Tier 2 – Non-Preferred Generic
- Tier 3 – Preferred Brand Name
- Tier 4 – Non-Preferred Brand Name Drugs
- Tier 5 – Specialty Drugs

There is also the *Famous Donut Hole*. To find out more, go to the Medicare Survival Guide Advanced edition, available at www.tonisays.com. As you are choosing a plan, it is critical to verify that your prescriptions are covered under that plan. If not, you need to be sure to find a plan that includes as many of your medications as possible.

If you are not going to take Medicare Part D, then you need to make sure that your current prescription plan is creditable and has been verified. These plans could include veterans' benefits or an employer/union group health plan. Social Security will allow you to delay enrolling in Medicare with a creditable prescription plan, but you need to make sure you have documented your previous coverage.

You have 63 days to enroll in a Medicare Part D prescription drug plan from a Creditable Prescription Coverage plan to keep from receiving a Part D penalty. Be sure that any verification forms for your creditable coverage are completed and kept up to date. Other parts of Medicare may have different deadlines, and it is important to track them to avoid missing critical deadlines that could negatively impact your coverage.

Now that you have a basic understanding of what each aspect of Medicare covers, and some critical points that you need, let's move on to Goalz 2: Understanding Medicare enrollment periods and how they can impact your enrollment process.

Goalz 4 U:

1. Medicare Part A is in-patient hospital coverage. skilled nursing and hospice

2. Medicare Part B is your medical coverage for outpatient surgery, doctor's visits, surgeons, durable medical equipment and more.

3. Medicare Part C is a Medicare Advantage plan, such as HMO, PPO, and other types of Medicare plans that help to cover what original Medicare does not.

4. Medicare Part D is Medicare prescription drug coverage.

Notes:

_____

_____

_____

_____

_____

_____

_____

_____

_____

_____

_____

_____

_____

_____

_____

_____

_____

GOALZ 2

Enrolling in
Medicare 4 U

Now that you are reaching 65, it is time to join the group called *Medicare beneficiaries*. You might be thinking that you don't need to enroll, because you already have medical coverage or since you are healthy and not currently dealing with any chronic medical conditions.

Just because that may be your situation, do not assume that you don't need to enroll in Medicare. By not doing so, you could end up costing yourself thousands of dollars in the years to come. How is that possible?

If you do not handle your enrollment correctly, you could end up joining another Medicare group: the ones who are paying lifetime penalties for their coverage. Currently, there are over 700,000 Medicare beneficiaries who are receiving a Medicare Part B and/or Part D penalty. These penalties are costing, on average, $5,000 in Medicare lifetime penalties. Why are the penalties so high?

Simply put, they did not enroll during their Medicare enrollment periods. Missing your enrollment period can cost you hundreds, if not thousands, of dollars. At the same time, there are plenty of people who will give you advice or tell you what you need to do. Do not listen to those individuals who want to tell you that you do not need to enroll or that you can just postpone enrollment until you are ready to retire.

Doing so puts you at risk of ending up with penalties, and those penalties can have a huge impact on your monthly retirement budget. Remember, these choices are going to play a role in how much of your fixed income is going to pay for your Medicare, and by taking the right steps during your enrollment, you can guarantee that you do not have to end up footing that expensive penalty bill.

Additionally, just because you are healthy, it does not mean that you are going to stay that way. You are taking a huge financial risk, because if you have something go wrong with your health, or even if you have to go to the doctor for a routine checkup, you put yourself in the position of being responsible for all the costs.

Let's get started by focusing on the various enrollment periods.

Toni Says®: Many believe that they do not need to enroll in Medicare when they are healthy and do not need a doctor. They are not aware of the Medicare Part B and Part D monthly penalty or No Part B or Part D coverage, and you will pay 100% for those benefits.

Medicare Initial Enrollment Period

Now, it would make the process much simpler if everyone had an enrollment period at the beginning of the year. Then, if you turned 65 during that year, you would be able to just enroll during that period, and your benefits would begin once you turned 65. However, this is the government, and rarely is anything that simple!

First, you need to understand that the government has defined your Initial Enrollment Period as beginning three months before the month that you turn 65, the month you turn 65, and then the three months after you turn 65. Essentially, you have a seven-month time frame to complete your enrollment without receiving any penalties.

Once you understand that time frame, it is now important that you understand that once you enroll, there may be a period of time before coverage starts. That time period will depend on when you enrolled.

It can be easy to assume that your coverage will begin immediately, but that is not the case. Let's talk about what you need to know regarding the start of coverage, which can help you to make the best choices regarding when you enroll.

When Does Your Initial Enrollment Period Begin?

If you enroll in Medicare during the three months prior to your birthday month, then your coverage will start the first day of your birthday month. Enrolling during this period also has the benefit of not having to worry about a physical or medical underwriting. You are going to be able to simply enroll and enjoy your Medicare coverage right from the time you turn 65, which is the best way to handle your enrollment.

Now, here is an important point to note. If your birthday lands on the 1st of the month, such as February 1, then your coverage will actually begin on January 1st. Simply put, being born on the first of the month means that you will have a month of coverage before you turn 65.

However, if you decide to wait until the month that you turn 65, or to use the three months after your birthday, then you will have your Medicare enrollment delayed. For the specific date that your coverage will start, then you need to talk with Social Security to determine what that day will be. The point is that by taking care of your enrollment early, you can avoid any penalties, while also enjoying your benefits for medical coverage and prescriptions (Medicare Part D).

Still, as long as you are covered by the end of your initial enrollment period, then you will not have to worry about penalties or medical underwriting. If you are delaying taking your Medicare Part B, there could be additional paperwork related to your enrollment period. However, you can claim a special enrollment period, which can keep you from being hit with penalties if you or your spouse are working full-time with true company benefits.

Additionally, it is important to know if you are going to take your Social Security or not. If you are not, then it will be your responsibility to connect with Social Security and get your enrollment started during your initial enrollment period. By not doing so, you put yourself at risk of a penalty.

Your Special Enrollment Period

If you decided to delay your Medicare Part B enrollment because you were covered by qualifying insurance, because you were working full-time with company benefits, or you were covered under your spouse's company benefits, then you can claim your Special Enrollment Period. If you are now going to stop working, then you will need to sign up for Medicare Part B within an eight-month window of your benefits ending.

If you are going to be covered by COBRA after you retire from your full-time job, then it is important to get your Medicare Part B enrollment started when your COBRA begins. Do not wait until your COBRA or company benefits are done, because it may be too late for you to claim your Medicare Part B benefits without a penalty.

Once that eight-month window passes, then you will be hit with penalties for every year that you were not enrolled in Medicare Part B prior to your enrollment. With those penalties, it can get quite expensive, as I have mentioned before. I cannot stress enough how important it is to pay attention to the dates. Getting distracted and not keeping track of critical dates can end up being very expensive.

Clearly, there are points that you need to consider before you arrive at your 65th birthday. Here are just a few to consider:

- What type of coverage are you getting at work?

- Are you still going to be working and able to access those benefits?

- If you are retiring, will you be taking your Social Security?

General Enrollment Period

If you opted not to enroll in Medicare Part B but did not have coverage to allow you to delay without penalty, you can take advantage of the General Enrollment Period from January 1st to March 31st, with your Medicare Part B beginning July 1st. Note that you will be able to enroll, but it will mean that you receive a Medicare Part B penalty. The size of this penalty will depend on each 12-month period you went without enrolling in Medicare Part B.

For instance, if you did not enroll in Medicare Part B until the general enrollment period in the year that you turn 70, you are going to have a large penalty, depending on how many 12-month periods you went without being enrolled in Medicare Part B. Needless to say, you are also going to have to deal with extensive medical underwriting and a prescription drug check, which can impact what Medicare advantage or supplement plans are available, and what you are going to pay for them.

As you can see, the first step to enrolling in Medicare is to understand the enrollment period options and how it can impact your finances throughout your retirement. I want you to not put yourself in the position of paying thousands into the system. Instead, I want you to do it right!

Now, let's start discussing the different scenarios that you might encounter during the enrollment process. We are going to walk you through the steps necessary to make sure that you are enrolled correctly.

At the end of each chapter, I am going to give you a short list of Goalz, those takeaways that you will need as part of your enrollment process. Let's get started!

Goalz 4 U

1. Initial Enrollment Period happens the year you turn 65, and starts three months before you turn 65, and ends three months after you turn 65.

2. Special Enrollment Periods are available if you delayed your Medicare Part B coverage because you had coverage through your company.

3. General Enrollment Period is from January 1st to March 31st, with your Medicare Part B beginning July 1st, and you must pay a penalty for your Medicare Part B or Part D for each 12-month period you went without Medicare Part B.

GOALZ 3

Enrolling in Medicare When Turning 65 and Receiving a Social Security Check

If you have tapped into your Social Security benefits, then you are going to find that the enrollment for Medicare is not going to be something that you must chase but will actually be one of the easiest and stress-free ways to receive your Medicare card. Why is this the case?

Social Security does all the paperwork for Medicare. With healthcare reform, the government has changed how they want you to enroll. So many things have become accessible online, and enrollment in Medicare is now one of them. Consider it a cost-saving measure of the government. Go to www.ssa.gov/benefits/medicare to begin the enrollment process if you are not already receiving your Social Security check. When you enroll online, it saves you hours in the Social Security office, plus it also saves you a lot of frustration in the process! (For more about enrolling online, go to Goalz 5.)

As I mentioned in the last chapter, knowing your enrollment period is key to successfully completing your online or in-office enrollment on time, and avoiding penalties. When you are claiming your Social Security, it makes the enrollment process more automatic, at least on the side of the government. Let's learn how.

Welcome to Medicare Kit

If you are already receiving your Social Security check, then you are going to receive a *Welcome to Medicare* kit in the mail. It will not only include information that you need as part of your enrollment process, but the packet will also include your new Medicare card.

Now, when you receive this packet, you are going to want to review everything in it, especially your new Medicare card. Make sure that the card includes both Medicare Parts A and B. If it doesn't, then you are not enrolled in any plan to cover your hospital, doctors, or other medical procedures. That lack of coverage could make you financially liable for any medical bills that you may receive once you turn 65.

If you do not receive your Medicare kit within that three-month period prior to your birthday month, then you need to be sure to contact Social Security. The reason that this is so important is because of that enrollment period. You have a limited window to enroll around your 65th birthday, and by delaying on your follow-up for your packet, you could be putting yourself at risk for penalties.

As part of your enrollment process, you will need to make sure that you enroll in Medicare Part A, B, and D. Doing so will help you to avoid any penalties for late enrollment. These parts are going to cover what you are likely going to use Medicare for during your retirement.

I mentioned earlier that this is the easiest and most stress-free way to enroll in Medicare.

What If I Am Not Drawing Social Security Just Yet?

If you are planning on drawing your Social Security at some point but have not yet started drawing that, then you might not receive your *Welcome to Medicare* kit prior to your 65th birthday. That can impact your enrollment period, so please check out Goalz 4 and 5, where I discuss this situation in depth, because it can have an impact on your enrollment period.

Recognize that there are going to be situations where you are not going to want to draw your Social Security due to your unique situation. You might still be working or might have opted to simply delay it to maximize your benefits. The point is that doing so will produce a situation where you will need to contact Social Security or go online and enroll in order to make sure you address the Medicare situation of enrolling in Medicare Part B properly.

Receiving VA Benefits and Social Security

There are several situations where you may be receiving Social Security but question whether you need to enroll in Medicare. One of those situations is if you are a veteran and currently receiving veteran's benefits. First, I want to thank you for your service to our nation. Second, you will still want to enroll in Medicare, even if you are receiving your veteran's benefits.

When you are a veteran receiving Social Security, then 90 days prior to turning 65, you will receive a *Welcome to Medicare* kit, along with your new Medicare card. On the back, it will state that you can sign the back to stop your Medicare Part B. Many vets have done this in the past, planning to claim it later, only to find themselves stuck with the famous 10% penalty per each 12-month period that they were not enrolled in Medicare. This penalty will last as long as the veteran is on Medicare Part B, or until the end of their lifetime.

Do not be quick to assume that because you are covered by the VA, you should just risk the potential penalty and stop your Medicare Part B. It could end up being more expensive than you realize in terms of medical costs that you have to cover if you end up needing services outside of the VA system and do not have the Medicare Part B. Plus, if you do enroll at a later date, that penalty can quickly add up.

For veterans, the VA provides specific benefits in response to their service to our country. I am the wife of a Vietnam Veteran, and the mother of two soldiers, and I am proud of their service. While it may seem as if the VA system is all you need, there may be instances when you need to get care and are not near the VA system, or you want to get in to see a doctor earlier than you can be accommodated by the VA system.

Having your Medicare Part B in place can help you in any cases where you want to step outside of the VA system for care. For instance, you might want to see a doctor outside of the VA network, which would be covered under Medicare enrollment. Another example is in the case of an emergency, where you would need to be seen quickly by someone outside of the VA network. Finally, there could be instances where you simply want to receive treatment closer to home, making having Medicare a helpful additional option to have.

How Part B Can Protect You as a Veteran

In Chapter 1, we discussed what Medicare Part B covers and some of the benefits of carrying Medicare Part B. It covers all your outpatient needs, doctor services, and even surgery. I haven't even scratched the surface of what is covered, or how you can use it to address your medical needs outside of the VA system.

Without that Medicare Part B enrollment, you could end up having to pay 100% out of your pocket for services associated with Medicare Part B, which could end up being thousands or even hundreds of thousands of dollars. I challenge you to look at your next bill outlining your medical services, and what those services cost the VA. Now, imagine if you had to pay those bills completely on your own. Scary, isn't it?

Here are a few other instances where not having Medicare Part B could come back to haunt you. A medical emergency might require that you be transported by ambulance to a hospital that is not part of the VA system. Without that Medicare Part B, you will incur all the costs associated with this ambulance ride, as well as any costs associated with treatment at that hospital. While you might be able to get reimbursement from the VA, you are still out the money until that reimbursement comes in.

Does this mean that you will never use your VA benefits? On the contrary, you will still be able to use those benefits to continue treatment or to address other issues as they come up. I also want to make it clear that having Medicare Part B does not mean that you are giving up your veterans' benefits. In fact, you are actually creating an additional layer of protection should you need it.

Another point to note is that you do not have to enroll in Medicare Part D. However, if you decide to enroll at a later date, you will not be penalized for your late enrollment in Medicare Part D because Medicare considers VA benefits as creditable coverage. I will be discussing creditable coverage in more detail throughout a number of different Goalz, so stay tuned!

As you can see, there are a variety of circumstances that you need to take into account when it comes to Medicare. Within this chapter, we have just scratched the surface. Our next few chapters are going to focus on situations that have far more complicated aspects, which can make it easier for you decide to enroll in Medicare Part B. I want to caution everyone that is thinking of delaying Medicare Part B, to be sure that you understand all the implications of your choice. It is critical to do it the right way, or risk penalties. You may also find that as you move forward, Medicare Part B is a better option than you thought.

The point of this chapter is that drawing Social Security makes Social Security's work simpler because you are automatically enrolled in Medicare when you turn 65. They do most of the work, and all you need to do is follow a few directions to make sure that you are enrolled. Now, let's move to a more complicated situation, one where you are not drawing your Social Security and you are self-employed, have an individual health plan, or have no health plan at all.

Goalz 4 U

1. By drawing Social Security at 65 or prior, due to various circumstances, you will receive a *Welcome to Medicare* kit, along with your Medicare card.

2. Check your card to make sure that both Medicare Part A and Part B are included.

3. Follow the enrollment process.

4. If you do not receive your packet, contact Social Security. Do not delay!

5. Retired Veterans should not delay Medicare Part B as Medicare can provide an additional layer of protection on top of their VA benefits. If you are a retired Veteran and you delay Medicare Part B and enroll at a later date you may receive the "famous" Medicare Part B penalty.

6. You will receive a Medicare Part B penalty if you or your spouse who covers you on their employer group health plan are not working full-time with true company benefits.

GOALZ 4

Turning 65, Not Receiving Social Security

While the process for enrolling in Medicare is fairly simple when you are already receiving Social Security or planning on taking your Social Security benefits once you turn 65, it can get more complicated if you are not opting to take your Social Security benefit at this time. Perhaps you are still working for yourself or are employed with an individual health plan. You might also be in a situation where you are working, but you have no employer group health benefits at all.

Like many Baby Boomers, you might be delaying receiving your Social Security check for a number of reasons. Perhaps you want to receive 100% of your benefits, and if you are still working, you might feel comfortable making that decision to wait. It can be easy to move through your 65th birthday without thinking about Medicare, because it is not even on your radar.

When you are self-employed, health care, and covering the costs associated with it, is your responsibility. You might have found yourself an individual health care plan or opted to just pay your health care costs as they come up. Now that you are getting older, however, you might be wondering if there is a way to reduce your out-of-pocket costs.

Clearly, there are multiple reasons why you should enroll in Medicare, with one of the biggest being to avoid the penalties that you can incur if you wait until you take your Social Security to enroll. However, since you are not taking Social Security, you will not be receiving any *Welcome to Medicare* kit from the Social Security office. Therefore, you are going to need to be proactive and start the process.

Enrolling in Medicare Without Receiving Your Social Security Check

Since Social Security is not going to know that you want to enroll, you will need to contact them 90 days before you turn 65. It is important that you do not delay on this, because your enrollment period is relatively small, and if you miss that window, then you run the risk of penalties.

If you wait until you are 65 to enroll in Medicare but not your Social Security check, you will need to go online to www.ssa.gov/benefits/medicare to begin enrolling. Visit Goalz 5 regarding enrolling in Medicare online. Do this within the 90-day window before turning 65.

Once you enroll, keep in mind that it will take Social Security about a week or so to process your paperwork. After the processing is complete, you will still have the same coverage start dates as I mentioned in Goalz 2, regarding enrollment periods. After you turn 65, you only have three more months before you are out of your Initial Enrollment Period.

Recognize that you cannot delay taking your Medicare Part B, because if you are self-employed and covered by an individual health care plan, that would not be deemed creditable health coverage for Medicare. Hence, you will incur a Medicare penalty if you decide not to enroll in Medicare Part B.

Recently, I worked with an individual who was self-employed and had been given some advice about delaying his enrollment in Medicare Part B. As I have said before, it is important to not listen to this well-meant advice. When you do, it can end up costing you a significant amount. For this individual, his Medicare nightmare is now starting, which is what might happen to you if you do not enroll in Medicare the correct way.

Why is Employer Group Health Coverage Important While Working?

Medicare does allow for delaying your Medicare Part B enrollment without penalties if you enroll later, but it involves having employer group health coverage through your or your spouse's employer. If you do not have insurance, then missing your enrollment period is going to mean that you are paying penalties. With that in mind, what does Medicare define as employer group health coverage?

Medicare recognizes true employer and union health plans with the Medicare recipient and/or their spouse **working full-time for that employer as qualified to delay Medicare.** If you are in this situation, then you are in the position where you can delay Medicare Part A and/or Part B for the working individual and their non-working spouse.

"COBRA and retiree health coverage do not count as current employer coverage," according to the *Medicare and You Handbook*. Essentially, if you have this type of health care coverage, you are not going to be able to delay your Medicare Part B. Most individual health plans, or not having health insurance benefits at all, are not going to fall under creditable coverage. Let me repeat: individual, COBRA and retirement health plans **are not current employer coverage** for those that are self-employed as you are, or retired.

Remember that individual I spoke of earlier that took their well-meaning friend's advice? He is self-employed, and now he is 66 years old. As a result of waiting to enroll in Medicare Part B, he is now going to receive a a 10% penalty per 12-month period that he could have had Medicare Part B but chose not to enroll or take it. His penalty will be a 20% penalty (two 12-month periods,

65 and 66) every month for as long as he is on Medicare. Essentially, he will be paying that penalty for the rest of his Medicare life.

Note that he is paying a penalty that goes back to when he could have enrolled when he turned 65. My advice is simple: make sure that you enroll during your enrollment period to avoid this financial hit later.

Your Initial Enrollment Period

Understand that your initial enrollment period spans over 7 months. You have 3 months before you turn 65, the month you turn 65, and then 3 months after you turn 65. As long as you get enrolled during this period, you will incur no 10% penalty for each 12-month period in which you could have enrolled and had Medicare Part B but failed to do so. I always encourage all Toni Says® clients to make sure that they have completed the Medicare enrollment process if they are not working full-time with employer group health benefits, or covered by their spouse that is working full-time with employer health benefits.

Not working full-time with true company benefits is what Medicare looks for, and it will incur the penalty. Recognize that if you are working full-time with company benefits, you are essentially able to delay your Medicare because you have employer group health coverage. However, if you happen to change jobs then, there is a paper trail that you need to create for Medicare, to avoid penalties.

A Working Spouse: Does It Matter?

At this point, the question comes up: what if I have a working spouse, and I get my coverage from them? If they are providing you with employer group health coverage, as I previously mentioned, then you may opt to delay enrolling in Medicare Part B.

If you do decide to follow this course, it is important that you create your paper trail for Medicare and Social Security, so that you do not incur a penalty when you do end up enrolling using your Special Enrollment Period. (For more about special enrollment periods, go to Goalz 1, where I discuss enrollment periods.)

You might continue to work either part-time or as a self-employed individual, taking advantage of the coverage provided by your spouse. I want to point out that some companies may ask you to enroll in Medicare once you are eligible, regardless whether your spouse continues to work for the company. Therefore, it is important to check with your spouse's human resources department to determine if you will still be able to carry coverage under your working spouse.

Do You Have Health Benefits?

If you are working full-time for yourself or someone else, you might still not be enjoying health benefits. In fact, you might be using an individual plan to provide coverage, or just living with no coverage at all.

Once your three-month enrollment period for Medicare begins prior to you turning 65, it is important to begin the enrollment process by going online at www.ssa.gov/benefits/medicare . There is no reason for you to miss out on this benefit or to pay for other health insurance coverage simply because you are not currently drawing Social Security.

Enrolling in Medicare the correct way when you are turning 65, or after 65, once you have retired from your company and are leaving your employer group health coverage, is key to avoiding penalties or risking having to cover medical costs out of your own pocket. Medicare does not accept the excuse that you didn't know. You do not get a second chance or a *do-over* when it comes to your Medicare enrollment period.

Talk with your spouse and determine whether you will be covered by your working spouse's medical insurance through work. If not, get enrolled. If you are self-employed or working at a job that does not provide coverage, then get enrolled. Next, I want to focus on how to enroll online. After all, many of us are used to using our computers or the internet for a variety of activities. By enrolling online, you can save yourself hours at the Social Security office, and have the ability to save critical paperwork right to your computer or online storage via the cloud. Let's get started!

Goalz 4 U

1. Know your Medicare enrollment period.

2. Determine if you have employer group health coverage and get the necessary documentation when delaying Medicare Part B and Part D enrollment, enrolling in Medicare at a later date when retiring, or leaving your or your spouse's employer group health plan.

3. Enroll in Medicare when turning 65 if you or your spouse are not working full-time, or if you are self-employed with individual coverage or no coverage at all.

4. Do not delay enrollment, as every 12-month period without enrollment incurs a 10% penalty per period, which will last throughout your lifetime.

Notes:

_____

_____

_____

_____

_____

_____

_____

_____

_____

_____

_____

_____

_____

_____

_____

_____

_____

GOALZ 5

Enrolling in Medicare Online When Turning 65

In a time of budget crunches, Social Security finally figured out that using technology could save them the cost of man-hours for Medicare enrollment. Two years ago, this plan was put into place, thus saving them payroll dollars, or should I say *our* tax dollars. What was this amazing plan of theirs? Simply put, they shifted the Medicare enrollment process to an online filing process. Now, when people turn 65, and they are not claiming their Social Security benefits, they can save themselves hours at the Social Security office by enrolling at www.ssa.gov/benefits/medicare.

Now, having read that first paragraph, you might be wondering what your Social Security check has to do with receiving your Medicare card. After all, I have been filing my taxes for years. Don't they know when I am turning 65? Why can't they just send me one of those *Welcome to Medicare* kits, regardless of whether I am claiming my Social Security benefits?

If you have reached 65 in the United States, then you should know that nothing with the U.S. government can be simple or easy. In fact, if there are unnecessary or cumbersome steps to be added to a process, the U.S. government is an expert at finding them and making sure that you must jump through all those loopholes to get the funding or benefits that you deserve.

Clearly, if nothing else is simple in dealing with the government, then why would Medicare enrollment be any different?

The Enrollment Process Online

Once you go to www.ssa.gov/benefits/medicare, you will be asked a few questions to help funnel you into the right slot, so to speak. The first key question is, "Do you have a *My Social Security* account?" If that is the case, then you will want to have your user name and password handy to begin your Medicare Part A and Part B application.

Now, if you do not have a *My Social Security* account, I want you to understand that starting one will not mean that you have claimed your Social Security benefits.

If you don't have a *My Social Security* account, then you need to complete the following:

- Please register yourself and your spouse for a *My Social Security* account, in the months before applying for Medicare, to be prepared for when you are ready to apply when turning 65 and need to apply for both Medicare Part A and Part B with an account, by visiting www.ssa.gov/myaccount.

- Part of the security process for registering for a *My Social Security* account involves being able to answer verification questions regarding you or your spouse's credit history. Don't worry if you aren't sure about an answer. This process can be confusing to many.

- If you are unable to open a *My Social Security* account by following the steps online, then you may need to contact Social Security, at 1-800-772-1213, or visit your local Social Security office for help.

- Call the Toni Says office, at 832-519-8664, or email info@ tonisays.com for assistance.

A word of advice before you get too frustrated: This system is not easy, and it has stumped even those with the highest levels of education under their belt. Don't hesitate to reach out for help to navigate the process. After all, if you don't get this right, it can impact your ability to enroll in Medicare, which could end up resulting in expensive penalties.

Not Receiving Your Social Security Check at 65

Unless you are receiving your Social Security check at least 90 days prior to turning 65, then Medicare has no idea you are turning 65. Why? Because Social Security, which handles all the enrollment for Medicare, does not know you are turning 65. Thus, Medicare has no idea that you should be receiving your Medicare card, with your Medicare Part A and Part B. Medicare does not enroll their own applications, because that whole process is done by Social Security.

As you can imagine, those who do not claim their Social Security benefits are simply ghosts to the Social Security department. You are not going to receive any information from Social Security about how to enroll. I am going to tell you now that this can be a huge Catch-22, one that ends up costing you a lot of money over the course of the rest of your life.

If you are opting not to receive your Social Security check, and you are not working full-time or covered under your working spouse's company benefits, then you are going to need to be proactive and enroll online through the Social Security website, www.ssa.gov/benefits/medicare; because, as I said earlier in this chapter, Social Security will not know that you are turning 65. However, if you or your spouse are working full-time and have true company benefits through that employer, it may be to your advantage to delay enrollment in Medicare Part A and B.

*The reason that you may want to delay your Medicare Part A enrollment when you turn 65 is because if you have an HSA, you will not be able to fund it once you are enrolled in Medicare Part A. That is because enrolling in Medicare Part A means that you are now enrolled in Medicare.

Social Security will advise you to enroll online if you call them, so the best thing you can do to protect yourself is to make a note to go to www.ssa.gov/benefits/medicare 90 days prior to the month that you turn 65. Doing so will mean that you are enrolled in Medicare Part A and Part B on the 1st day of the month that you turn 65. That coverage will be available to you as you turn 65.

Now, I want to share with you the steps that you need to follow in order to make sure that you have covered everything necessary for your enrollment. Doing so will make sure that you are not hit with a penalty at a later date for missing key enrollment steps.

I also want to point out that if you are getting ready to turn 65 in the next month or so, you still have time to complete your enrollment without dealing with a late penalty for Medicare Part B. The importance of not delaying is something that I cannot stress enough. When it comes to any interactions with the government, not knowing about a deadline is no excuse and will not help you to avoid penalties. Medicare enrollment is no different.

What If I Can't Open My Social Security Account?

If you are not able to open a *My Social Security* account when turning 65, you can still move forward with the sign-up for Medicare. Click on the **EXIT** button and proceed to the Medicare sign-up page. This information cannot be found anywhere in any Social Security information on *How to Enroll in Medicare*. If you cannot proceed with applying for Medicare without opening a *My Social Security* account, then what?

Go directly to your local Social Security office and inform the Social Security agent that you are not able to open a Social Security account, and that you need assistance. Remember that Social Security is using online enrollment as a budget saving measure, but keep in mind that they still keep agents to help if you run into trouble.

Once you have a *My Social Security* account, then you need to open the Medicare sign-up page and start imputing the information that is requested. Here are a few pieces that you need to have:

- Begin with your information: Name, Social Security number, gender, and date of birth.

- Contact information, which should include your address, phone number, and email address.

- Citizen information, including what language you read and speak.

- If you are a naturalized citizen, you may need to bring your citizenship paperwork to Social Security.

- There will be questions regarding your health benefits.

After you complete the online application, hit the submit button. Then you begin the process of waiting for your benefits verification letter to arrive. As with so many things that need to come from the government, there is going to be a waiting game. I cannot stress enough that you need to get these items taken care of right away, because natural government delays could mean that you run out of time to address any issues, which could increase the potential for penalties.

Once your new Medicare card arrives, make sure that it includes Medicare Part A and Part B. If it doesn't, you need to contact Social Security right away. However, if both Medicare Part A and Part B are on your card, then you may want to enroll in a Medicare Supplement Plan, along with a stand-alone Medicare Part D prescription drug plan, or enroll in a Medicare Advantage Plan with a prescription drug plan, to help pick up the medical costs that Medicare does not pay for.

If you are not enrolled in Medicare Part A or B, you will not be able to enroll in a Medicare Supplement or Advantage Plan and a Medicare Part D Prescription Plan. If you do not enroll in a Medicare Part D Prescription Drug Plan, then you risk penalties for not enrolling during your initial enrollment period.

As you can see, the process of enrolling in Medicare can be complicated, so be sure to start the process early. Now I want to shift your focus to Goalz related to those who do have company health benefits once they turn 65. In Goalz 6, I want to focus on what you need to do if you or your spouse are still working full-time but enroll in Medicare Part A and Part B.

Goalz 4 U:

1. Starting a *My Social Security* account does not mean that you are claiming your Social Security benefits.

2. Put your username and password for your *My Social Security* account in a safe place, because you will need it in the future, both

for your Medicare enrollment and for checking on your Social Security benefits in the future.

3. Remember, if you cannot open up a *My Social Security* account to enroll in Medicare, and are locked out because you could not answer your credit questions, or maybe your Social Security account is locked due to someone hacking your credit, then click the **EXIT** button, and you should be taken directly to the Medicare application.

4. If you cannot start a *My Social Security* **account**, or have issues getting into the Medicare application, then contact Social Security, at 1-800-772-1213, or go to your local Social Security office and ask for help.

Notes:

_____

_____

_____

_____

_____

_____

_____

_____

_____

_____

_____

_____

_____

_____

GOALZ 6

Turning 65 with Company Benefits

In Goalz 3 and 4, I was focused on enrolling in Medicare during your seven-month Initial Enrollment Period, which includes the three months prior to you turning 65, the month that you are turning 65, and the three months after you turn 65. In Goalz 6, I will explain what happens if you are still working full-time and enroll in Medicare Parts A and B.

There are three scenarios that can come into play if you are still working when you turn 65. I am going to outline each of them and how it can impact your enrollment. Every day, I talk with someone who gets the wrong information from a well-meaning friend. With all that often-conflicting advice from individuals who are not experts in enrolling in Medicare, it can be easy to make critical errors that leave you on the hook for penalties and other issues.

As for Medicare not educating folks about their rules, please don't get me started on that one! I mentioned before that Medicare has provided special rules for those who could fall under the category of *still working* with true company benefits and turning 65.

One of the most important things to remember is that true company benefits have a rather narrow definition. Time and again, I see individuals who might have medical coverage under their retirement benefits, or coverage through COBRA, and they make the mistake in thinking that those are true company benefits. Please remember that there is not an "oops!" clause in Medicare if you make a mistake in this area. Penalties will still kick in later, even if you thought you were able to delay Medicare enrollment due to having medical coverage through another source. Let's get started by looking at each scenario and what you need to know.

Scenario #1 – Turning 65, Social Security Benefits, True Company Benefits

Scenario #1 – Turning 65, receiving your Social Security check with true company benefits from your work, or you may also have true company benefits if you are covered under your working spouse's company benefits. Clearly, you have medical coverage, and you may be wondering if you should keep or delay your Medicare? If you decide to delay your Medicare, the question is, how can you do so to avoid any potential penalties?

Let me introduce you to Sam. He began to get his Social Security benefits at 62. Sam has always been on his wife's company benefits. When he turned 65, Medicare sent him his Medicare card with Medicare Parts A and B, with an effective date starting the 1ˢᵗ of the month that he turned 65. Sam now has a decision to make when he turns 65.

First, Sam could opt to delay his Medicare Part B for a later date and apply for Medicare Part B when his spouse retires with a SEP (Special Enrollment Period), which is discussed in Goalz 7. On the back of the Medicare card, Sam could simply sign in the spot where it states that he would like to delay his Medicare Part B for a later date, and then mail it back to Social Security. Doing so would mean that he would not have his Medicare premium deducted from his Social Security check.

During a Medicare consultation, I always advise my clients who are delaying Medicare Part B to find out how the employer medical claims will be paid. One of the reasons for this is that while Sam may want to delay his Medicare Part B for a later date, it can also delay his Medicare Supplement/Medigap Open Enrollment period. This enrollment period is six-months long and starts the day that Medicare Part B begins. If you delay, then you will be able to enroll in your Medicare supplement coverage without having to answer one underwriting question.

The Medicare Supplement/Medigap Open Enrollment period only happens when one has first started their Medicare Part B for the first time, whether turning 65 or past 65.

Now, Sam could opt to enroll in his Medicare Part B and remain covered under his wife's company benefits as well. However, once she retires, he then will have to answer medical questions to enroll in any Medicare Supplement. The reason is that he has been enrolled in his Medicare Part B longer than 6 months and will be past the Medicare Supplement/Medicare Open Enrollment period. If he currently has mild medical conditions, this might not be a concern, but for those that are dealing with medical issues, having to answer those medical questions could impact what a supplemental plan costs, or the ability to even be approved in a Medicare Supplement plan at all.

As you can see, Sam has choices to make, and those decisions can impact his costs and options in the future.

Scenario #2 – Turning 65, No Social Security Benefits, True Company Benefits (Your or Your Spouse's Employer)

Scenario #2 – In this scenario, you have opted to continue working full-time and are not claiming your Social Security benefits. This situation could also involve your spouse continuing to work full-time with true company benefits.

For Sally, she is now working full-time and has true company benefits. She is not retiring at 65, and does not plan on taking her Social Security benefits. Sally is concerned about applying for Medicare because she has received numerous calls from telemarketers that are confusing her. They are telling her that she has to enroll in Medicare, because if she does not, then she will get the dreaded Medicare Part B and Part D penalties.

Does she have the option of delaying her Medicare Part B and D without penalties if she has true company benefits under her employer or her spouse's employer?

Let's find out together...

In the *Medicare and You* handbook, it states: "If you or your spouse are covered under employer benefits, it may be to your advantage to delay your Medicare Part B for a later date. You will apply during your Special Enrollment Period (SEP)." (See Goalz 7 about *Applying for Medicare Past 65 with Employer Benefits*)

There are rules to make sure that your delay is documented so that you can take advantage of the SEP. What if you are not the one working full-time? Does that make a difference?

According to Medicare, if you have true company benefits under your spouse's employer, you have the same option to delay your Medicare Part B and D enrollment, just as Sally did.

Another scenario, to add to Scenario #2, is Jerry's, whose spouse is covered under his employer's group benefits, so the same Medicare rule will apply for them as it did for Sally. Namely, Jerry and his spouse will need to apply for a Special Enrollment Period (SEP) if they are past 65 and 90 days, just like Sally, when leaving Jerry's company benefits or retiring.

Scenario #3 – 65, No Social Security Benefits

In this scenario, there are true company benefits in place, but those benefits are coming with a significant cost. What are the options for this individual?

Sidney is turning 65 and has true company benefits. He has opted to not take his Social Security benefits at this time, but his company benefits have a high deductible with a large monthly premium, which is killing his paycheck. He currently has very few prescriptions, and Sidney is wondering if enrolling in Medicare Part B and D might be a better alternative.

Sidney needs to study Goalz 5, and then he can follow those steps to enroll in Medicare within the 90 days of the month he turns 65, in order for his Medicare to begin on the 1st day of his 65th birthday month, during his Medicare Initial Enrollment period. During this Initial Enrollment period, Sidney also can enroll in a Medicare Supplement Plan, along with a Medicare stand-alone Part D plan, a zip code specific Medicare Advantage Plan, or Original Medicare only, with a stand-alone Medicare Part D plan.

If Sidney does have prescriptions, which are expensive and can get him in the *famous Donut Hole*, then he may not want to apply for Medicare until he retires, especially if he is covered under employer group benefits that are creditable as far as prescriptions are concerned. (Check out Chapter 1 regarding the various Medicare Parts, for an understanding of what the *Donut Hole* is.)

Essentially, if you find yourself in a situation where you have costly prescriptions, then you might find that delaying Medicare enrollment is the better option to minimize your prescription out-of-pocket costs. You can then wait until you retire and receive a SEP (Special Enrollment Period) form that shows you were covered with true company benefits during the time that you were not enrolled in Medicare but were eligible. (See Goalz 7 for more information.)

As you can see, there are several different scenarios that can come into play if you are still working and receiving true company benefits. Depending on what the company benefits are, and what your out-of-pocket is, you may find that enrolling in Medicare may be a more cost-effective option. Keep in mind that if your company funds an HSA, however, enrolling in Medicare will essentially stop them from doing so. If the reimbursement amount for your HSA is significant, that may be something else that you want to factor into your decision.

Goalz 4 U:

1. If you are working full-time and have true company benefits under your employer or a spouse's employer, then you may delay your enrollment in Medicare Part B and Part D.

2. If you are delaying your Medicare Part D coverage, then it is important to make sure that your company's prescription drug plan falls under the creditable coverage as defined by Medicare.

3. If you are working full-time with true company benefits, you may still enroll in Medicare Parts A and B, but you will have to answer medical underwriting questions when applying for a Medicare

Supplement past the 6-month Medicare Supplement/Medigap Open Enrollment period. It is very important to understand this Medicare rule.

4. If you decide to delay your Medicare enrollment, you will need to get a Special Enrollment Period (SEP) form to enroll in Medicare Part B and Part D without penalty. (See Goalz 7)

Notes:

_____

_____

_____

_____

_____

_____

_____

_____

_____

_____

_____

_____

_____

_____

_____

_____

GOALZ 7

Past 65 and 90 Days:
Magic Words...
"Is Still Working"

When it comes to avoiding penalties for Medicare Part B, it is important to know the magic words: *"is still working."* These magic words are critical when it comes to enrolling in Medicare past 65 and you or your spouse are losing company benefits.

The *Medicare and You Handbook*, under the title of *Should I Enroll in Medicare Part B*, discusses delaying Medicare Part B when you are leaving your or your spouse's group benefits. "You can sign up for Medicare Part B anytime during the 8-month period that begins the month after the employment ends or the coverage ends, whichever happens first," says the *Medicare and You Handbook*.

When I perform a Medicare planning consultation at the Toni Says® office, whether just laid off or retiring, I stress the value of getting Medicare Part B for the first time, and that Medicare Part B needs to be enrolled in prior to either enrolling in COBRA or retirement group benefits, because of continuation of coverage rules that want to coordinate with Medicare.

You have 8-months to enroll in Medicare Parts A and Part B once you or your spouse are not working full-time, without receiving the famous *Medicare Part B penalty*. At the Toni Says office, during a Medicare consultation, I advise those no longer working full-time to have their Medicare Part B in place the 1st of the month that they are not employed. The 8-month window is there for your protection to not receive the Medicare Part B penalty that goes back to the 1st of the month that your Medicare began, or you turned 65.

The forms listed below must be signed by your HR or benefits manager, for you and/or your spouse, who have been covered through company benefits since turning 65 and are now wishing to enroll in Medicare Part B and refrain from receiving the famous *Part B penalty*.

There are 2 forms available from Social Security's website, or you can ask for them from the Toni Says® office (info@tonisays.com). On the top of each form, write in *red letters, "Special Enrollment Period."* This tells the Social Security agent that is processing them that you are signing up at the right time, and it keeps you from getting a penalty. You are applying for a **SEP (Special Enrollment Period).**

- **Form #1 Request for Employment Information Social Security form # CMS-L564:** proof of group health care coverage based on current employment. If you have had 2 or more jobs since turning 65, then all companies you or your spouse have worked for, from age 65 to the time you or your spouse are retiring, are to sign this form. If you are married, you will need the same number of forms filled out for your non-working spouse, and signed by the companies' HR departments for which you or your spouse had worked, proving the non-working spouse was covered by company insurance (if the non-working spouse is Medicare or Medicare eligible). On the top of each form, write in *red letters, "Special Enrollment Period."*

- **Form #2 Application for Enrollment in Medicare Part B form # CMS-40-B:** this is you and your spouse's application for medical insurance from Medicare, known as Part B. Social Security fills out this form. Also, on the top of each form, write in *red letters, "Special Enrollment Period."*

The above forms are to be used for all who are asking for a Special Enrollment Period due to leaving company benefits past 65, and who want to avoid the famous *Medicare Part B penalty.*

A healthcare professional once told me that many of the newest healthcare and cancer procedures are not readily approved by insurance plans, and that these procedures are generally approved with *Original or Traditional Medicare*. He said he must fight the insurance companies every day to get his patients the care they desperately need. Do not put yourself in this position by not enrolling in a timely fashion for Medicare Part B.

The process to receiving a SEP and enrolling in Medicare Part A and/or B past 65, as mentioned above, is the same whether you or your spouse are leaving company benefits because of:

1. Health issues, since Medicare will pay for the specific procedure you need, that your company benefits will not cover.

2. You have been laid off, as many companies are laying off their high-income earners, and that seems to be those who are past 65.

3. You have decided to retire.

Goalz 4 U:

1. Always have Part B in place when leaving your job or losing your company benefits. Do not wait!

2. Fill out the *Request for Employment Information* Social Security form # CMS-L564 to avoid the penalty for late enrollment in Medicare Part B, when leaving company group health benefits after turning 65.

3. Even though Medicare gives an 8-month period to avoid the famous *Medicare Part B penalty*…Do not wait, but have your

Medicare Part B begin the 1st of the month when you or your spouse are no longer working full-time.

4. Enroll in Medicare Parts A and B when receiving COBRA benefits, to avoid paying Medicare's Part B penalty and extra Medicare costs.

GOALZ 8

Turning or Past 65 Receiving COBRA Benefits

Americans, especially those turning 65, do not realize how important it is to enroll the right way for Medicare Part B and Part D. In fact, because they have been working, it might never have crossed their minds to even start looking at Medicare enrollment.

Now that many of these same individuals are now leaving their jobs or losing them after they turn 65, Medicare enrollment comes as a gigantic surprise.

This is particularly the case when they enroll in Medicare Part B after being on COBRA. For those who come into the Toni Says® office for a Medicare consultation regarding their Medicare Part B and Part D benefits, we stress how important it is to make sure that your Medicare coverage starts the day your company benefits end, or the day your COBRA plan starts.

Why is This So Important?

In the *Medicare and You Handbook*, under "Should I Get Part B?" it discusses the rules of COBRA and their impact on your Medicare eligibility or late penalties. I have talked to many individuals who thought that their Special Enrollment Period (SEP) starts when their COBRA ends in 18 months. Instead, they find themselves facing late penalties, which start from the month they were eligible to enroll in Medicare until the day they do enroll.

As I mentioned in earlier Goalz, those penalties can be costly, and they will last for the rest of your lifetime. I want you to be aware of the fact that most Americans simply do not know about these penalties, but it can impact them for years to come.

Simply put, you need to understand that your Special Enrollment Period (SEP) begins the month you lose your company benefits or when your employment ends, whichever comes first. You might have gone on COBRA, but COBRA is not considered true company benefits by Medicare.

Hence, if you decide to take COBRA, and wait until it ends to enroll in Medicare Part B, you are going to face the late enrollment penalties, plus you are at risk of having to deal with the medical questionnaires as well, which can impact your Medicare Part C options and how much you pay for them.

Those that think COBRA is the same as company benefits are often in for a BIG SURPRISE. Once they enroll in Medicare Part B, they are finding they are penalized 10% each year or 12-month period they could have had Part B but didn't. The penalty goes all the way back to the day he/she turned 65.

Case in Point: The 14-Year Penalty

To illustrate how expensive this can become, I want to illustrate it with a client of mine. He lived in Wharton, TX, and was 79 years old. For many years, he was on his wife's company health plan, so he never enrolled in Medicare Part B. She was the working spouse, but she ended up losing her job. She was 62 at the time and had health issues of her own. After looking at Heathcare.gov, she realized that COBRA was the less expensive option, so she enrolled both of them on a COBRA plan. I bet you all can already see the mistake that they made.

When COBRA finally ended for both of them 18 months later, they went to the Social Security office to enroll her husband in Medicare Part B. They were shocked by what they heard!

My client's premium for his Medicare Part B in the year they enrolled was $134.00. Keep in mind, the premiums are subject to change each year. Now it was time to access his penalty. You can probably do the math. You take 79-65, which equals 14 years. Now, this elderly gentleman is facing a 10% penalty per 12-month period that he could have had Medicare Part B but chose not to enroll or take it. He has fourteen 12-month periods, which is 10% times 14. That is a 140% penalty that lasts the rest of his life! That year, his penalty was $187.60 (10% of that year's Medicare Part B monthly premium times fourteen 12-month periods). His total monthly Medicare Part B premium, with penalty, is now $134 + $187.60 = $321.60 per month for that year.

Keep in mind that this amount would only apply for that year. If the monthly premiums increase the next year, then his penalty is going to increase as well. Did you notice that his penalty was actually more than the cost of his premium? Now, imagine how much more budget friendly that would have been for them if he only had to worry about that premium. Instead, that penalty of 140% is going to be a monthly expense for the rest of his Medicare life.

I cannot stress enough how important it is to enroll in Medicare Part B at the right time. When you do not, it can end up being a costly mistake that will haunt your retirement finances for the rest of your life.

What About Your COBRA?

You might find yourself in a similar position. It might be that you planned on working longer, and that you have enjoyed true company benefits throughout your employment. If you refer back to Goalz 7, then you will find out what you need to do in order to delay your Medicare Part B benefits without a penalty.

However, you cannot assume that your Special Enrollment Period (SEP) begins when your COBRA ends. I want to stress it again that COBRA is not true company benefits. If you find yourself suddenly losing your job or being forced to retire due to an unexpected health crisis, you might be tempted to push enrollment in Medicare Part B off until after your COBRA ends. Do not do this!

You may find well-meaning individuals from your HR department might tell you that you do not need to enroll in Medicare just yet. Do not believe them! As soon as you know you are losing your company benefits, then you need to make sure that you start the Medicare enrollment process. Be sure to write "Special Enrollment Period (SEP)," in red, on the top of your Social Security form, Request for Employment Information, to make sure that you do not have the penalty.

Remember, so many Americans think that the Medicare Part B rule only starts when COBRA ends in 18 months. They are not aware that the Special Enrollment Period (SEP) begins the month they lose their company benefits or that their employment ends—essentially, when they go onto COBRA.

I do not want you to end up dealing with sticker shock, like so many other Americans, either due to a spouse's Medicare enrollment or your own. Just so you know, arguing with Social Security is a wasted effort. "Them's the Rules," and Social Security does not make exceptions. Simply put, Medicare and Social Security do not recognize COBRA as health coverage based on current employment or true company benefits.

Goalz 4 U:

1. Always have Medicare Part B in place when leaving your job or losing your company benefits. DO NOT WAIT!!

2. As part of your Special Enrollment Period, which begins when your company benefits or your employment ends, make sure you have the Social Security form, Request for Employment Information, signed by your HR department, which shows you have had true company benefits between the time that you turned 65 and the time you are no longer working full-time and lost your company benefits.

Notes:

_____

_____

_____

_____

_____

_____

_____

_____

_____

_____

_____

_____

_____

_____

_____

_____

GOALZ 9

Medicare Forms for SEP & Lowering Medicare Part B and Part D Premiums

Throughout this guide, my focus has been on helping you to understand key aspects of enrollment, and dispelling the idea that you can enroll in Medicare at any time after you turn 65. The truth is that you have an Initial Enrollment Period (IEP) when turning 65, a Special Enrollment Period (SEP) when past 65 and leaving company group health benefits, and General Enrollment Period (GEP) when past 65 and not working full-time with company group health benefits and applying for Medicare for the first time.

Therefore, it is important to make sure that you are staying on top of the dates around the time that you turn 65, especially if you are not taking your Social Security benefits at that time. Unless you have true company benefits through your employer or your spouse's employer, you will not be able to delay Medicare Part B and Part D enrollment without late penalties.

In this Goalz, I wanted to give you a picture of what these forms look like, so you can be sure that you are completing the right ones and avoiding a mistake that could end up costing you in terms of penalties.

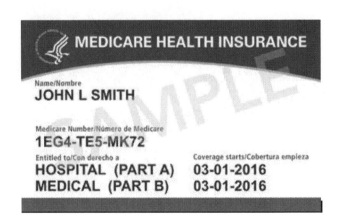

DEPARTMENT OF HEALTH AND HUMAN SERVICES
CENTERS FOR MEDICARE & MEDICAID SERVICES

Form Approved
OMB No. 0938-0787

REQUEST FOR EMPLOYMENT INFORMATION

WHAT IS THE PURPOSE OF THIS FORM?

In order to apply for Medicare in a Special Enrollment Period, you must have or had group health plan coverage within the last 8 months through your or your spouse's current employment. People with disabilities must have large group health plan coverage based on your, your spouse's or a family member's current employment.

This form is used for proof of group health care coverage based on current employment. This information is needed to process your Medicare enrollment application.

The employer that provides the group health plan coverage completes the information about your health care coverage and dates of employment.

HOW IS THE FORM COMPLETED?

- Complete the first section of the form so that the employer can find and complete the information about your coverage and the employment of the person through which you have that health coverage.
- The employer fills in the information in the second section and signs at the bottom.

WHAT DO I DO WITH THE FORM?

Fill out Section A and take the form to your employer. Ask your employer to fill out Section B. You need to get the completed form from your employer and include it with your Application for Enrollment in Medicare (CMS-40B). Then you send both together to your local Social Security office. Find your local office here: **www.ssa.gov**.

GET HELP WITH THIS FORM

- **Phone:** Call Social Security at **1-800-772-1213**
- **En español:** Llame a SSA gratis al **1-800-772-1213** y oprima el 2 si desea el servicio en español y espere a que le atienda un agente.
- **In person:** Your local Social Security office. For an office near you check **www.ssa.gov**.

DEPARTMENT OF HEALTH AND HUMAN SERVICES
CENTERS FOR MEDICARE & MEDICAID SERVICES

Form Approved
OMB No. 0938-0787

REQUEST FOR EMPLOYMENT INFORMATION

SECTION A: To be completed by individual signing up for Medicare Part B (Medical Insurance)

1. Employer's Name

2. Date

3. Employer's Address

City

State

Zip Code

4. Applicant's Name

5. Applicant's Social Security Number

6. Employee's Name

7. Employee's Social Security Number

SECTION B: To be completed by Employers

For Employer Group Health Plans ONLY:

1. Is (or was) the applicant covered under an employer group health plan? ☐ Yes ☐ No

2. If yes, give the date the applicant's coverage began. (mm/yyyy)

3. Has the coverage ended? ☐ Yes ☐ No

4. If yes, give the date the coverage ended. (mm/yyyy)

5. When did the employee work for your company?

From: (mm/yyyy)

To: (mm/yyyy)

Still Employed: (mm/yyyy)

6. If you're a large group health plan and the applicant is disabled, please list the timeframe (all months) that your group health plan was primary payer.

From: (mm/yyyy)

To: (mm/yyyy)

For Hours Bank Arrangements ONLY:

1. Is (or was) the applicant covered under an Hours Bank Arrangement? ☐ Yes ☐ No

2. If yes, does the applicant have hours remaining in reserve? ☐ Yes ☐ No

3. Date reserve hours ended or will be used? (mm/yyyy)

All Employers:

Signature of Company Official

Date Signed

Title of Company Official

Phone Number

( ) –

According to the Paperwork Reduction Act of 1995, no persons are required to respond to a collection of information unless it displays a valid OMB control number. The valid OMB control number for this information is 0938-0787. The time required to complete this information collection is estimated to average 15 minutes per response, including the time to review instructions, search existing data resources, gather the data needed, and complete and review the information collection. If you have comments concerning the accuracy of the time estimate(s) or suggestions for improving this form, please write to: CMS, 7500 Security Boulevard, Attn: PRA Reports Clearance Officer, Mail Stop C4-26-05, Baltimore, MD 21244-1850.

Form CMS-L564 (CMS-R-297) (09/16)

2

Form Approved
OMB No. 0938-0787

STEP BY STEP INSTRUCTIONS FOR THIS FORM

SECTION A:

The person applying for Medicare completes all of Section A.

1. **Employer's name:**
   Write the name of your employer.

2. **Date:**
   Write the date that you're filling out the Request for Employment Information form.

3. **Employer's address:**
   Write your employer's address.

4. **Applicant's Name:**
   Write your name here.

5. **Applicant's Social Security Number:**
   Write your Social Security Number here.

6. **Employee's Name:**
   If you get group health plan coverage based on your employment, write your name here. If you get group health plan coverage through another person, like a spouse or family member, write their name.

7. **Employee's Social Security Number:**
   If you get group health plan coverage based on your employment, write your Social Security Number here. If you get group health plan coverage through another person, like a spouse or family member, write their Social Security Number.

Once you complete Section A:

Once Section A is completed, give this form to your employer to complete Section B. Once Section B has been completed by your employer, return this form along with your Part B application to your local Social Security office.

SECTION B:

The employer completes all of Section B.

If you're an employer without an hours bank arrangement, complete the section called "For Employer Group Health Plans ONLY"

1. **Is (or was) the applicant covered under an employer group health plan?**
   Please check yes or no if the applicant was covered under your group health plan offered by your company. The applicant may be the employee or another person related to the employee, such as a spouse or family member with disabilities. If your company doesn't offer a group health plan, please check No. A group health plan is any plan of one or more employers to provide health benefits or medical care (directly or otherwise) to current or former employees, the employer, or their families.

2. **If yes, give the date the coverage began.**
   Write the month and year the date the applicant's coverage began in your group health plan.

3. **Has the coverage ended?**
   Check yes or no if the group health plan coverage for the applicant has ended.

4. **If yes, give the date the coverage ended.**
   Write the month and year the group health plan coverage ended for the applicant.

5. **When did the employee work for your company?**
   Write the start and end dates of the employment for the employee in which the applicant is related. It may be the applicant or another person related to the employee, such as a spouse or family member with disabilities.

   Enter the month and year of the start of the employment in the "From" box.

   Enter the month and year of end of the employment in the "To" box.

   If the employee is still employed, enter the month and year of the current date.

   Current employment is active working status. It is not disability or retirement.

6. **If you're a large group health plan and the applicant is disabled, please list the timeframe (all months) that your group health plan was primary payer.**
   Write the start and end dates that your group health plan was primary payer for the applicant.

If you're an employer with an hours bank arrangement, complete the section called "For Hours Bank Arrangements ONLY"

1. **Is (or was) the applicant covered under an hours bank arrangement?**
   Please check yes or no if the applicant was covered under an hours bank arrangement. If you check no, please also fill out the section for "Employer Group Health Plans ONLY".

2. **If yes, does the applicant have hours remaining in reserve?**
   Please indicate if the applicant currently has health coverage based on the remaining hours in the employee's hours bank account.

3. **Date reserve hours ended or will be used?**
   Please write the month and year for when the remaining hours in the employee's hours bank account expired or will expire.

All employers need to complete the bottom of Section B.

- **Signature of Company Official:**
  An official representative of the company needs to sign this document. Please do not print.

- **Date Signed:**
  Write the date that you sign the form in this field.

- **Title of Company Official:**
  Print the title of the company official who signed the form in this field.

- **Phone Number:**
  Write the phone number of the company official who signed the form in this field. If there are questions regarding the information on this form, a representative from Social Security will contact you.

DEPARTMENT OF HEALTH AND HUMAN SERVICES
CENTERS FOR MEDICARE & MEDICAID SERVICES

Form Approved
OMB No. 0938-1230
Expires: 02/20

APPLICATION FOR ENROLLMENT IN MEDICARE PART B (MEDICAL INSURANCE)

WHO CAN USE THIS APPLICATION?
People with Medicare who have Part A but not Part B

NOTE: If you do **not** have Part A, do **not** complete this form. Contact Social Security if you want to apply for Medicare for the first time.

WHEN DO YOU USE THIS APPLICATION?
Use this form:
- If you're in your **Initial Enrollment Period** (IEP) and live in **Puerto Rico**. You must sign up for Part B using this form.
- If you're in your **IEP** and **refused Part B** or did not sign up when you applied for Medicare, but now want Part B.
- If you want to sign up for Part B during the General Enrollment Period (GEP) from January 1 – March 31 each year.
- If you refused Part B during your IEP because you had group health plan (GHP) coverage through your or your spouse's current employment. You may sign up during your 8-month Special Enrollment Period (SEP).
- If you have Medicare due to disability and refused Part B during your IEP because you had group health plan coverage through your, your spouse or family member's current employment.
- You may sign up during your 8-month SEP.

NOTE: Your IEP lasts for 7 months. It begins 3 months before your 65th birthday (or 25th month of disability) and ends 3 months after you reach 65 (or 3 months after the 25th month of disability).

WHAT INFORMATION DO YOU NEED TO COMPLETE THIS APPLICATION?
You will need:
- Your Medicare Number
- Your current address and phone number
- Form CMS-L564 "Request for Employment Information" completed by your employer **if you're signing up in a SEP**.

WHAT HAPPENS NEXT?
Send your completed and signed application to your local Social Security office. If you sign up in a SEP, include the CMS-L564 with your Part B application. If you have questions, call Social Security at **1-800-772-1213**. **TTY users should call 1-800-325-0778.**

HOW DO YOU GET HELP WITH THIS APPLICATION?
- **Phone:** Call Social Security at **1-800-772-1213**. TTY users should call **1-800-325-0778**.
- **En español:** Llame a SSA gratis al **1-800-772-1213** y oprima el 2 si desea el servicio en español y espere a que le atienda un agente.
- **In person:** Your local Social Security office. For an office near you check **www.ssa.gov**.

REMINDERS
- If you sign up for Part B, you must pay premiums for every month you have the coverage.
- If you sign up after your IEP, you may have to pay a late enrollment penalty (LEP) of 10% for each full 12-month period you don't have Part B but were eligible to sign up.

CMS-40B (04/18)

1

DEPARTMENT OF HEALTH AND HUMAN SERVICES
CENTERS FOR MEDICARE & MEDICAID SERVICES

Form Approved
OMB No. 0938-1230
Expires: 02/20

APPLICATION FOR ENROLLMENT IN MEDICARE PART B (MEDICAL INSURANCE)

1. Your Medicare Number

2. Do you wish to sign up for Medicare Part B (Medical Insurance)? ☐ YES

3. Your Name (Last Name, First Name, Middle Name)

4. Mailing Address (Number and Street, P.O. Box, or Route)

5. City

State

Zip Code

6. Phone Number (including area code)

(　　　)　　　　–　　　　

7. Written Signature (DO NOT PRINT)

SIGN HERE

8. Date Signed

　　/　　/　　

**IF THIS APPLICATION HAS BEEN SIGNED BY MARK (X), A WITNESS WHO KNOWS THE APPLICANT
MUST SUPPLY THE INFORMATION REQUESTED BELOW.**

9. Signature of Witness

10. Date Signed

　　/　　/　　

11. Address of Witness

12. Remarks

According to the Paperwork Reduction Act of 1995, no persons are required to respond to a collection of information unless it displays a valid OMB control number. The valid OMB control number for this information collection is 0938-1230. The time required to complete this information is estimated to average 15 minutes per response, including the time to review instructions, search existing data resources, gather the data needed, and complete and review the information collection. If you have any comments concerning the accuracy of the time estimate(s) or suggestions for improving this form, please write to: CMS, Attn: PRA Reports Clearance Officer, 7500 Security Boulevard, Baltimore, Maryland 21244-1850.

CMS-40B (04/18)

2

Form Approved
OMB No. 0938-1230
Expires: 02/20

SPECIAL MESSAGE FOR INDIVIDUAL APPLYING FOR PART B

This form is your application for Medicare Part B (Medical Insurance). You can use this form to sign up for Part B:

- During your Initial Enrollment Period (IEP) when you're first eligible for Medicare
- During the General Enrollment Period (GEP) from January 1 through March 31 of each year
- If you're eligible for a Special Enrollment Period (SEP), like if you're covered under a group health plan (GHP) based on current employment.

Initial Enrollment Period

Your IEP is the first chance you have to sign up for Part B. It lasts for 7 months. It begins 3 months before the month you reach 65, and it ends 3 months after you reach 65. If you have Medicare due to disability, your IEP begins 3 months before the 25th month of getting Social Security Disability benefits, and it ends 3 months after the 25th month of getting Social Security Disability benefits. To have Part B coverage start the month you're 65 (or the 25th month of disability insurance benefits); you must sign up in the first 3 months of your IEP. If you sign up in any of the remaining 4 months, your Part B coverage will start later.

General Enrollment Period

If you don't sign up for Part B during your IEP, you can sign up during the GEP. The GEP runs from January 1 through March 31 of each year. If you sign up during a GEP, your Part B coverage begins July 1 of that year. You may have to pay a late enrollment penalty if you sign up during the GEP. The cost of your Part B premium will go up 10% for each 12-month period that you could have had Part B but didn't sign up. You may have to pay this late enrollment penalty as long as you have Part B coverage.

Special Enrollment Period

If you don't sign up for Part B during your IEP, you can sign up without a late enrollment penalty during a Special Enrollment Period (SEP). If you think that you may be eligible for a SEP, please contact Social Security at 1-800-772-1213. TTY users should call 1-800-325-0778 You can use a SEP when your IEP has ended. The most common SEPs apply to the working aged, disabled, and international volunteers.

Working Aged/Disabled

You have a SEP if you're covered under a group health plan (GHP) based on **current** employment. To use this SEP, you must:

- Be 65 or older and currently employed
- Be the spouse of an employed person, and covered under your spouse's employer GHP based on his/her current employment
- Be under 65 and disabled, and covered under a GHP based on your own or your spouse's current employment

You can sign up for Part B anytime while you have a GHP coverage based on current employment or during the 8 months after either the coverage ends or the employment ends, whichever happens first. If you sign up while you have GHP coverage based on current employment, or, during the first full month that you no longer have this coverage, your Part B coverage will begin the first day of the month you sign up. You can also choose to have your coverage begin with any of the following 3 months. If you sign up during any of the remaining 7 months of your SEP, your Part B coverage will begin the month after you sign up.

NOTE: COBRA coverage or a retiree health plan is not considered group health plan coverage based on current employment.

International Volunteers

You have a SEP if you were volunteering outside of the United States for at least 12 months for a tax-exempt organization and had health insurance (through the organization) that provided coverage for the duration of the volunteer service.

Privacy Act Statement: Social Security is authorized to collect your information under sections 1836, 1840, and 1872 of the Social Security Act, as amended (42 U.S.C. 1395o, 1395s, and 1395ii) for your enrollment in Medicare Part B. Social Security and the Centers for Medicare & Medicaid Services (CMS) need your information to determine if you're entitled to Part B. While you don't have to give your information, failure to give all or part of the information requested on this form could delay your application for enrollment. Social Security and CMS will use your information to enroll you in Part B. Your information may be also be used to administer Social Security or CMS programs or other programs that coordinate with Social Security or CMS to:

1) Determine your rights to Social Security benefits and/or Medicare coverage.
2) Comply with Federal laws requiring Social Security and CMS records (like to the Government Accountability Office and the Veterans Administration)
3) Assist with research and audit activities necessary to protect integrity and improve Social Security and CMS programs (like to the Bureau of the Census and contractors of Social Security and CMS). We may verify your information using computer matches that help administer Social Security and CMS programs in accordance with the Computer Matching and Privacy Protection Act of 1988 (P.L. 100-503).

CMS-40B (04/18)   3

Form Approved
OMB No. 0938-1230
Expires: 02/20

STEP BY STEP INSTRUCTIONS FOR FILLING OUT THIS APPLICATION

1. **Your Medicare Number:**
   Write your Medicare number.

2. **Do you wish to sign up for Medicare Part B (Medical Insurance)?**
   Mark "YES" in this field if you want to sign up for Medicare Part B which provides you with medical insurance under Medicare. You can only sign up using this form if you already have Medicare Part A (Hospital Insurance). If your answer to this question is "no" then you don't need to fill out this application. This application is to sign up to get medical insurance under Medicare.

   If you don't have Part A and want to sign up, please contact Social Security at 1-800-772-1213. TTY users should call 1-800-325-0778.

3. **Name:**
   Write your name as you did when you applied for Social Security or Medicare. List last name, first name and middle name in that order. If you don't have a middle name, leave it blank.

4. **Mailing Address:**
   Write your full mailing address including the number and street name, P.O. Box, or route in this field.

5. **City, State, and ZIP code:**
   Write the city name, state and ZIP code for the mailing address.

6. **Phone Number:**
   Write your 10-digit phone number, including area code.

7. **Written Signature:**
   Sign your name in this section in the same way you would sign it for any other official document. Do not print.

   If you're unable to sign, you may mark an "X" in this field. In this case, you will need a witness and the witness must complete questions 11, 12 and 13.

8. **Date Signed:**
   Write the date that you signed the application.

9. **Signature of Witness:**
   In the case that question 9 is signed by an "X" instead of a written signature, a witness signature is needed in question 11 showing that the person who signs the application is the person represented on the application.

10. **Date Signed:**
    If a witness signs this application, the witness must provide the date of the signature.

11. **Address of Witness:**
    If a witness signs this application, provide the witness's address.

12. **Remarks:**
    Provide any remarks or comments on the form to clarify information about your enrollment application.

IMPORTANT INFORMATION:

Review the scenario below to determine if you need to include additional information or forms with your application.

If you're signing up for Part B using a Special Enrollment Period (SEP) because you were covered under a group health plan based on current employment, in addition to this application, you will also need to have your employer fill and return the "Request for Employment Information" form (**CMS-L564/CMS-R-297**) with your application. The purpose of this form is to provide documentation to Social Security that proves that you have been continuously covered by a group health plan based on current employment, with no more than 8 consecutive months of not having coverage. If your employer went out of business or refuses to complete the form, please contact Social Security about other information you may be able to provide to process your SEP enrollment request.

Send the application (and the "Request for Employment Information," if applicable) to your local Social Security Office. Find your local office at **www.ssa.gov**.

Form **SSA-44** (12-2018)
Discontinue Prior Editions
Social Security Administration

Medicare Income-Related Monthly Adjustment Amount - Life-Changing Event

If you had a major life-changing event and your income has gone down, you may use this form to request a reduction in your income-related monthly adjustment amount. See page 5 for detailed information and line-by-line instructions. If you prefer to schedule an interview with your local Social Security office, call 1-800-772-1213 (TTY 1-800-325-0778).

Name	Social Security Number

You may use this form if you received a notice that your monthly Medicare Part B (medical insurance) or prescription drug coverage premiums include an income-related monthly adjustment amount (IRMAA) and you experienced a life-changing event that may reduce your IRMAA. To decide your IRMAA, we asked the Internal Revenue Service (IRS) about your adjusted gross income plus certain tax-exempt income which we call "modified adjusted gross income" or MAGI from the Federal income tax return you filed for tax year 2017. If that was not available, we asked for your tax return information for 2016. We took this information and used the table below to decide your income-related monthly adjustment amount.

The table below shows the income-related monthly adjustment amounts for Medicare premiums based on your tax filing status and income. If your MAGI was lower than $85,000.01 (or lower than $170,000.01 if you filed your taxes with the filing status of married, filing jointly) in your most recent filed tax return, you do not have to pay any income-related monthly adjustment amount. If you do not have to pay an income-related monthly adjustment amount, you should not fill out this form even if you experienced a life-changing event.

If you filed your taxes as:	And your MAGI was:	Your Part B monthly adjustment is:	Your prescription drug coverage monthly adjustment is:
-Single, -Head of household, -Qualifying widow(er) with dependent child, or -Married filing separately (and you did not live with your spouse in tax year)*	$ 85,000.01 - $107,000.00 $107,000.01 - $133,500.00 $133,500.01 - $160,000.00 $160,000.01 - $500,000.00 More than $500,000.00	$ 54.10 $135.40 $216.70 $297.90 $325.00	$ 12.40 $ 31.90 $ 51.40 $ 70.90 $ 77.40
-Married, filing jointly	$170,000.01 - $214,000.00 $214,000.01 - $267,000.00 $267,000.01 - $320,000.00 $320,000.01 - $750,000.00 More than $750,000.00	$ 54.10 $135.40 $216.70 $297.90 $325.00	$ 12.40 $ 31.90 $ 51.40 $ 70.90 $ 77.40
-Married, filing separately (and you lived with your spouse during part of that tax year)*	$85,000.00 - $415,000.00 More than $415,000.00	$297.70 $325.00	$ 70.90 $ 77.40

* Let us know if your tax filing status for the tax year was Married, filing separately, but you lived apart from your spouse at all times during that tax year.

STEP 1: Type of Life-Changing Event

Check **ONE** life-changing event and fill in the date that the event occurred (mm/dd/yyyy). If you had more than one life-changing event, please call Social Security at 1-800-772-1213 (TTY 1-800-325-0778).

☐ Marriage   ☐ Work Reduction

☐ Divorce/Annulment   ☐ Loss of Income-Producing Property

☐ Death of Your Spouse   ☐ Loss of Pension Income

☐ Work Stoppage   ☐ Employer Settlement Payment

Date of life-changing event: _____

mm/dd/yyyy

STEP 2: Reduction in Income

Fill in the tax year in which your income was reduced by the life-changing event (see instructions on page 6), the amount of your adjusted gross income (AGI, as used on line 37 of IRS form 1040) and tax-exempt interest income (as used on line 8b of IRS form 1040), and your tax filing status.

Tax Year	Adjusted Gross Income	Tax-Exempt Interest
2 0 __ __	$ __ __ __ __ __ . __ __	$ __ __ __ __ __ . __ __

Tax Filing Status for this Tax Year (choose **ONE**):

☐ Single   ☐ Head of Household   ☐ Qualifying Widow(er) with Dependent Child

☐ Married, Filing Jointly   ☐ Married, Filing Separately

STEP 3: Modified Adjusted Gross Income

Will your modified adjusted gross income be lower next year than the year in Step 2?

☐ No - Skip to STEP 4

☐ Yes - Complete the blocks below for next year

Tax Year	Estimated Adjusted Gross Income	Estimated Tax-Exempt Interest
2 0 __ __	$ __ __ __ __ __ . __ __	$ __ __ __ __ __ . __ __

Expected Tax Filing Status for this Tax Year (choose **ONE**):

☐ Single   ☐ Head of Household   ☐ Qualifying Widow(er) with Dependent Child

☐ Married, Filing Jointly   ☐ Married, Filing Separately

STEP 4: Documentation

Provide evidence of your modified adjusted gross income (MAGI) and your life-changing event. You can either:

1. Attach the required evidence and we will mail your original documents or certified copies back to you;

OR

2. Show your original documents or certified copies of evidence of your life-changing event and modified adjusted gross income to an SSA employee.

Note: You must sign in Step 5 and attach all required evidence. Make sure that you provide your current address and a phone number so that we can contact you if we have any questions about your request.

STEP 5: Signature

PLEASE READ THE FOLLOWING INFORMATION CAREFULLY BEFORE SIGNING THIS FORM.

I understand that the Social Security Administration (SSA) will check my statements with records from the Internal Revenue Service to make sure the determination is correct.

I declare under penalty of perjury that I have examined the information on this form and it is true and correct to the best of my knowledge.

I understand that signing this form does not constitute a request for SSA to use more recent tax year information unless it is accompanied by:

• Evidence that I have had the life-changing event indicated on this form;
• A copy of my Federal tax return; or
• Other evidence of the more recent tax year's modified adjusted gross income.

Signature	Phone Number	
Mailing Address	**Apartment Number**	
City	**State**	**ZIP Code**

93

THE PRIVACY ACT

We are required by sections 1839(i) and 1860D-13 of the Social Security Act to ask you to give us the information on this form. This information is needed to determine if you qualify for a reduction in your monthly Medicare Part B and/or prescription drug coverage income-related monthly adjustment amount (IRMAA). In order for us to determine if you qualify, we need to evaluate information that you provide to us about your modified adjusted gross income. Although the responses are voluntary, if you do not provide the requested information we will not be able to consider a reduction in your IRMAA.

We rarely use the information you supply for any purpose other than for determining a potential reduction in IRMAA. However, the law sometimes requires us to give out the facts on this form without your consent. We may release this information to another Federal, State, or local government agency to assist us in determining your eligibility for a reduction in your IRMAA, if Federal law requires that we do so, or to do the research and audits needed to administer or improve our efforts for the Medicare program.

We may also use the information you provide in computer matching programs. Matching programs compare our records with records kept by other Federal, state or local government agencies. We will also compare the information you give us to your tax return records maintained by the IRS. The law allows us to do this even if you do not agree to it. Information from these matching programs can be used to establish or verify a person's eligibility for Federally funded or administered benefit programs and for repayment of payments or delinquent debts under these programs.

Explanations about these and other reasons why information you provide us may be used or given out are available in Systems of Records Notice 60-0321 (Medicare Database File). The Notice, additional information about this form, and any other information regarding our systems and programs, are available on-line at www.socialsecurity.gov or at your local Social Security office.

Paperwork Reduction Act Statement - This information collection meets the requirements of 44 U.S.C. § 3507, as amended by section 2 of the Paperwork Reduction Act of 1995. You do not need to answer these questions unless we display a valid Office of Management and Budget control number. We estimate that it will take about 45 minutes to read the instructions, gather the facts, and answer the questions. **SEND OR BRING THE COMPLETED FORM TO YOUR LOCAL SOCIAL SECURITY OFFICE. The office is listed under U. S. Government agencies in your telephone directory or you may call Social Security at 1-800-772-1213 (TTY 1-800-325-0778).** *You may send comments on our time estimate above to: SSA, 6401 Security Blvd, Baltimore, MD 21235-6401.* **Send *only* comments relating to our time estimate to this address, not the completed form.**

INSTRUCTIONS FOR COMPLETING FORM SSA-44
Medicare Income-Related Monthly Adjustment Amount
Life-Changing Event--Request for Use of More Recent Tax Year Information

You do not have to complete this form in order to ask that we use your information about your modified adjusted gross income for a more recent tax year. If you prefer, you may call 1-800-772-1213 and speak to a representative from 7 a.m. until 7 p.m. on business days to request an appointment at one of our field offices. If you are hearing-impaired, you may call our TTY number, 1-800-325-0778.

Identifying Information

Print your full name and your own Social Security Number as they appear on your Social Security card. Your Social Security Number may be different from the number on your Medicare card.

STEP 1

You should choose only one life-changing event on the list. If you experienced more than one life-changing event, please call your local Social Security office at 1-800-772-1213 (TTY 1-800-325-0778). Fill in the date that the life-changing event occurred. The life-changing event date must be in the same year or an earlier year than the tax year you ask us to use to decide your income-related premium adjustment. For example, if we used your 2015 tax information to determine your income-related monthly adjustment amount for 2017, you can request that we use your 2016 tax information instead if you experienced a reduction in your income in 2016 due to a life-changing event that occurred in 2016 or an earlier year.

Life-Changing Event	Use this category if...
Marriage	You entered into a legal marriage.
Divorce/Annulment	Your legal marriage ended, and you will not file a joint return with your spouse for the year.
Death of Your Spouse	Your spouse died.
Work Stoppage or Reduction	You or your spouse stopped working or reduced the hours that you work.
Loss of Income-Producing Property	You or your spouse experienced a loss of income-producing property that was not at your direction (e.g., not due to the sale or transfer of the property). This includes loss of real property in a Presidentially or Gubernatorially-declared disaster area, destruction of livestock or crops due to natural disaster or disease, or loss of property due to arson, or loss of investment property due to fraud or theft.
Loss of Pension Income	You or your spouse experienced a scheduled cessation, termination, or reorganization of an employer's pension plan.
Employer Settlement Payment	You or your spouse receive a settlement from an employer or former employer because of the employer's bankruptcy or reorganization.

INSTRUCTIONS FOR COMPLETING FORM SSA-44

STEP 2

Supply information about the more recent year's modified adjusted gross income (MAGI). Note that this year must reflect a reduction in your income due to the life-changing event you listed in Step 1. A change in your tax filing status due to the life-changing event might also reduce your income-related monthly adjustment amount. Your MAGI is your adjusted gross income as used on line 37 of IRS form 1040 plus your tax-exempt interest income as used on line 8b of IRS form 1040. We used your MAGI and your tax filing status to determine your income-related monthly adjustment amount.

Tax Year

- Fill in both empty spaces in the box that says "20_ _". The year you choose must be more recent than the year of the tax return information we used. The letter that we sent you tells you what tax year we used.

  - Choose this year (the "premium year") - if your modified adjusted gross income is lower this year than last year. For example, if you request that we adjust your income-related premium for 2019, use your estimate of your 2018 MAGI if:

    1. Your income was not reduced until 2019; or
    2. Your income was reduced in 2018, but will be lower in 2019.

  - Choose last year (the year before the "premium year," which is the year for which you want us to adjust your IRMAA) - if your MAGI is not lower this year than last year. For example, if you request that we adjust your 2019 income-related monthly adjustment amounts and your income was reduced in 2018 by a life-changing event AND will be no lower in 2019, use your tax information for 2018.

  - Exception: If we used IRS information about your MAGI 3 years before the premium year, you may ask us to use information from 2 years before the premium year. For example, if we used your income tax return for 2016 to decide your 2019 IRMAA, you can ask us to use your 2017 information.

- If you have any questions about what year you should use, you should call SSA.

Adjusted Gross Income

- Fill in your actual or estimated adjusted gross income for the year you wrote in the "tax year" box. Adjusted gross income is the amount on line 37 of IRS form 1040. If you are providing an estimate, your estimate should be what you expect to enter on your tax return for that year.

Tax-exempt Interest Income

- Fill in your actual or estimated tax-exempt interest income for the tax year you wrote in the "tax year" box. Tax-exempt interest income is the amount reported on line 8b of IRS form 1040. If you are providing an estimate, your estimate should be what you expect to enter on your tax return for that year.

Filing Status

- Check the box in front of your actual or expected tax filing status for the year you wrote in the "tax year" box.

INSTRUCTIONS FOR COMPLETING FORM SSA-44

STEP 3

Complete this step only if you expect that your MAGI for next year will be even lower and will reduce your IRMAA below what you told us in Step 2 using the table on page 1. We will record this information and use it next year to determine your Medicare income-related monthly adjustment amounts. If you do not complete Step 3, we will use the information from Step 2 next year to determine your income-related monthly adjustment amounts, unless one of the conditions described in "Important Facts" on page 8 occurs.

Tax Year

- Fill in both empty spaces in the box that says "20 _ _ " with the year following the year you wrote in Step 2. For example, if you wrote "2019" in Step 2, then write "2020" in Step 3.

Adjusted Gross Income

- Fill in your estimated adjusted gross income for the year you wrote in the "tax year" box. Adjusted gross income is the amount you expect to enter on line 37 of IRS form 1040 when you file your tax return for that year.

Tax-exempt Interest Income

- Fill in your estimated tax-exempt interest income for the tax year you wrote in the "tax year" box. Tax-exempt interest income is the amount you expect to report on line 8b of IRS form 1040.

Filing Status

- Check the box in front of your expected tax filing status for the year you wrote in the "tax year" box.

STEP 4

Provide your required evidence of your MAGI and your life-changing event.

Modified Adjusted Gross Income Evidence

If you have filed your Federal income tax return for the year you wrote in Step 2, then you must provide us with your signed copy of your tax return or a transcript from IRS. If you provided an estimate in Step 2, you must show us a signed copy of your tax return when you file your Federal income tax return for that year.

Life-Changing Event Evidence

We must see original documents or certified copies of evidence that the life-changing event occurred. Required evidence is described on the next page. In some cases, we may be able to accept another type of evidence if you do not have a preferred document listed on the next page. Ask a Social Security representative to explain what documents can be accepted.

Life-Changing Event	Evidence
Marriage	An original marriage certificate; or a certified copy of a public record of marriage.
Divorce/Annulment	A certified copy of the decree of divorce or annulment.
Death of Your Spouse	A certified copy of a death certificate, certified copy of the public record of death, or a certified copy of a coroner's certificate.
Work Stoppage or Reduction	An original signed statement from your employer; copies of pay stubs; original or certified documents that show a transfer of your business. **Note:** In the absence of such proof, we will accept your signed statement, under penalty of perjury, on this form, that you partially or fully stopped working or accepted a job with reduced compensation.
Loss of Income-Producing Property	An original copy of an insurance company adjuster's statement of loss or a letter from a State or Federal government about the uncompensated loss. If the loss was due to investment fraud (theft), we also require proof of conviction for the theft, such as a court document citing theft or fraud relating to you or your spouse's loss.
Loss of Pension Income	A letter or statement from your pension fund administrator that explains the reduction or termination of your benefits.
Employer Settlement Payment	A letter from the employer stating the settlement terms of the bankruptcy court and how it affects you or your spouse.

STEP 5

Read the information above the signature line, and sign the form. Fill in your phone number and current mailing address. It is very important that we have this information so that we can contact you if we have any questions about your request.

Important Facts

• When we use your estimated MAGI information to make a decision about your income-related monthly adjustment amount, we will later check with the IRS to verify your report.

• If you provide an estimate of your MAGI rather than a copy of your Federal tax return, we will ask you to provide a copy of your tax return when you file your taxes.

• If your estimate of your MAGI changes, or you amend your tax return for that reason, you will need to contact us to update our records. If you do not contact us, we may have to make corrections later including retroactive assessments or refunds.

• We will use your estimate provided in Step 2 to make a decision about the amount of your income-related monthly adjustment amounts the following year until:

  • IRS sends us your tax return information for the year used in Step 2; or
  • You provide a signed copy of your filed Federal income tax return or amended Federal income tax return with a different amount; or
  • You provide an updated estimate.

• If we used information from IRS about a tax year when your filing status was Married filing separately, but you lived apart from your spouse at all times during that year, you should contact us at 1-800-772-1213 (TTY 1-800-325-0778) to explain that you lived apart from your spouse. Do not use this form to report this change.

These forms are just one piece of the puzzle during the enrollment process. Working with the Toni Says® office, we can help you to understand what you need to know about the enrollment process and also how Medicare Advantage Part C enrollment works. I encourage you to contact us for a consultation if you have any questions regarding the enrollment process and what your different Medicare options can be. Waiting can end up costing you more than you realize!

Notes:

_____

_____

_____

_____

_____

_____

_____

_____

_____

_____

_____

_____

_____

_____

_____

_____

_____

GOALZ 10

Enrolling is Just the Beginning

Throughout this guide, I have attempted to share the situations that I have run across most frequently in my role as a Medicare consultant. Along the way, I am reminded about how much false or misleading information is out there. Even the most well-meaning friends and family members are going to give you advice or information that is, at best, partially inaccurate, and at worst, completely false. It can end up costing you in terms of premiums, penalties, and even out-of-pocket costs down the road.

Clearly, there is a lot more going on than most people realize. Turning 65 has turned into a birthday that you cannot let slide by without addressing your Medicare situation. For years, working adults have assumed that if they kept working, then they didn't need to worry about Medicare. It has become a symbol of retirement, something that more and more of us are putting off until we are much older.

However, that is simply not the case. Medicare is tied to your 65th birthday, whether you are still going to work or have decided to retire. Do not make the mistake that so many have, of waiting until they retire to address their Medicare enrollment. Using this guide is the first step to helping you through the enrollment process and to avoid critical and expensive pitfalls.

Now that I have given you the tools to make it through the Medicare enrollment process, I realized that it gets even more complicated from here. After all, just because you managed to avoid the late enrollment penalties or having to do a medical questionnaire does not mean you are in the clear yet. In fact, there are now more decisions to make. You are going to have to decide what type of supplement coverage you want, or if an advantage plan will serve you better.

I have run into so many individuals who are confused about what Medicare options are, and which Medicare option best meets their medical and financial needs at that specific time and for the future. Plus, you have the added confusion of multiple ads running constantly around Medicare's open enrollment, claiming that they can help you find the best deal for your budget. It can make the process of determining fact from fiction very complicated, to say the least.

Part of the reason that I wrote my original Medicare Survival Guide Advanced, was that I wanted to share key points to help you throughout Medicare, giving you the information to navigate this complicated government process. Due to changes in the rules of Medicare, I have updated my Medicare Survival Guide Advanced, creating the current edition, available at the store, at www.tonisays.com. If you haven't already picked it up, I encourage you to do so. It can give you a variety of information about Medicare, based on real life experiences from people just like you.

At this point, you might be wondering if it is possible to navigate this process without costing yourself in terms of coverage or premium pricing. This government program is complicated, and it can trip up anyone. I cannot stress enough the importance of doing your homework and making sure that you have the right information. It means doing your due diligence and finding a consultant who can help to walk you through the process.

Part of what the Toni Says® team does is assist people through the enrollment process. We work to answer their questions and help them understand the information that they are receiving from Social Security. Too often, individuals fail to realize that if they do not have written documentation, but only verbal information, you essentially have nothing for backup. Social

Security is never wrong, and without written documentation, you cannot argue with them effectively.

I would encourage you to make sure that you have copies of all your Medicare information from Social Security, including the enrollment process. Make a backup copy that you keep somewhere offsite, in case your home is lost due to fire or a natural disaster.

The reason I bring this up is that many states have faced an increase in natural disaster events, including fires and flooding. Homes have been completely lost, including valuable papers, such as Social Security cards, birth certificates, and more. While much of that paperwork can be replaced, your correspondence with Social Security regarding your Medicare enrollment cannot be replaced.

There are also technological backup options that you can explore, such as cloud backup and scans saved on a drive and put in a safety deposit box. There are many more options available today than just a firebox in your home. I encourage you to explore your options to make sure that you have all your backup.

The Goalz 4 U at the end of each of these chapters are meant to help you understand what you need to do, depending on your unique situation. If you are not sure your situation is covered in this guide, then contact me at info@Tonisays.com, and I can help answer your questions. With years of experience navigating the Medicare system, I have the knowledge that can help you to get through the process.

Along the way, I plan on adding more Goalz 4 U guides regarding various aspects of the Medicare process. If there is something you want to know more about, then message me at info@Tonisays.com. I want to hear from you, because your experiences are a large part of why I do what I do.

Too many of my clients have come to me after they turn 65, struggling to understand what they need to do now. If you take nothing else away from this guide, I want you to take away that without coverage from true company benefits, either through your job or your spouse's, then you need to get enrolled in Medicare.

In the meantime, I wish you the best Medicare journey as you continue working or enter your retirement. May the journey be an amazing adventure, and may this guide help make your journey with Medicare smoother.

Goalz 4 U:

1. Get the Medicare Survival Guide Advanced, edition, to explore your Medicare options, available at www.tonisays.com.

2. Contact ToniSays.com® with any questions, or to take advantage of our Medicare consulting services, at info@tonisays.com, or call 832-519-8664.

About the Author

Toni King is an author, columnist, and radio and TV personality, and has spent more than 27 years as a top sales leader in the Medicare and health insurance fields. She has also conducted "Confused about Medicare" workshops, throughout Texas and the southeastern United States.

In 2008, Toni was holding a Medicare workshop in Greenville, Mississippi, when a member of the audience asked a question about his not needing Medicare Part B. Toni met with the gentleman after the workshop, and it didn't take her long to find out that he had received wrong information from his local Social Security office. It took a couple of days to get this overwhelming problem straightened out and get him his Medicare Part B. When it was all finished, her role as an insurance agent had changed to that of advocate for people on Medicare. It was then that she took the <u>Medicare and You</u> handbook, and put it into *people terms*, so the average person could understand Medicare.

Whether Toni is consulting with a client in the office, or giving a "Confused about Medicare" workshop to hundreds of people, she emphasizes her mottos: *Medicare is NOT Cookie-Cutter*, and *What You Don't Know WILL Hurt You!* Not understanding the rules and guidelines of Medicare can cause you to make costly mistakes that will last a lifetime. Whether you are helping your parents understand Medicare or choosing a plan for yourself, let Toni show you how to navigate your way through what has become the Medicare maze!

Toni King lives in Houston, TX, with her husband of 26 years, Jim King, and has two sons. Both sons have served in the military. John served in the army in Iraq and Afghanistan, and Michael in the Marine Corps stateside. Jim is a decorated Vietnam veteran, who served in the Marine Corps. Toni often says she bleeds "red, white, and blue."

Made in the
USA
Lexington, KY